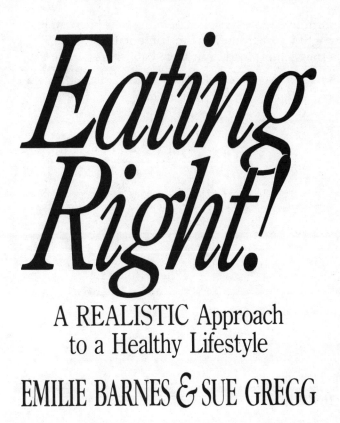

Eating Right!

A REALISTIC Approach to a Healthy Lifestyle

EMILIE BARNES & SUE GREGG

HARVEST HOUSE PUBLISHERS
Eugene, Oregon 97402

EATING RIGHT!

Copyright © 1987 by Harvest House Publishers
Eugene, Oregon 97402

Library of Congress Catalog Card Number 87-081037
ISBN 0-89081-613-1

Printed in the United States of America.

To our husbands, Bob Barnes and Rich Gregg,
who have eaten everything in this book
and whose patience, support, and encouragement
have made this book possible,
and to the families who have found and will find
a new Eating Better Lifestyle.

CONTENTS

Part 4—Nitty Gritty Nutrition News

Part 5—Biblical Perspectives

Part 6—Action

Part 7—Appendix

Menu and Recipe Index

MENUS

RECIPES

Meatless Main Dishes

1

Emilie's Story

As busy women we plan (or do not plan), shop, prepare, and cook over 750 meals per year. That is a major part of our lives. As I've been teaching More Hours In My Day seminars, one of the most frequently asked questions is "Where can I get ideas on balanced, nutritious meal planning, especially for my dinner meals?" We get into a rut with meals and need new, fresh ideas.

Fast-food restaurants are now preparing meals for us. For example, one major fast-food restaurant sells a triple cheese-burger with over 1,200 calories. Being overweight is a major problem for many people. Fad diets and diet books are best-sellers, and new fad diets pop up daily in magazines, news-papers, and books. How can we balance our health, weight, and the dilemma of the busy woman's meal planning? The answer is on the way!

First, though, let me tell you how it all began.

A Friday morning Bible study started when our son's best friend, Todd Miller, a 16-year-old professional motocross racer, was killed at the national championship race in Ana-heim, California. Bob and Elaine's only child, gone. Tragedy and grief filled our neighborhood. Several of the neighbor-hood women suggested we start a support group Bible study in my home to help Elaine through the loss of Todd. Up to 50 women attended with as many as 28 children in the nursery. God truly blessed as our lives were changed.

I'll never forget the first Friday morning that Sue Gregg came. A friend brought her. Two weeks earlier, Sue's three-year-old son, Stephen, was killed in the Greggs' front yard by a drunken teenaged driver. Sue shared her story that day. We were blessed by Sue's testimony of comfort and peace in the loss of her son.

Not long after coming to the Bible study, Sue attended one of my seminars. When I shared a short segment on proper foods and eating nature's way, I demonstrated the difference in size between a loaf of white bread and a loaf of whole wheat bread by squeezing each from end to end. Sue's eyes lit up. A simple demonstration triggered her interest. God began a new work in her that day.

Now, let me go even further back.

My father, Otto Klein, was born and orphaned at a very early age in Vienna, Austria. At that time many European countries would place the orphans in areas where they could learn a vocation. My father had the wonderful opportunity of being placed in the kitchen in the Palace of Vienna where he worked side by side with some of the most famous chefs in the world. When he came as a young man to America, he came as a very fine Viennese chef. As the supervising chef he opened many fine hotels and restaurants in the United States. In later years he worked for the movie studios and cooked for national and international celebrities.

My father cooked only with real butter, olive oil, and the very best natural ingredients. He always used brown rice and fresh vegetables. Ketchup and canned or frozen foods were a disgrace. He would receive compliments and standing ovations for his cooking. His secret was using high-grade natural ingredients with creative flair and quality perfection.

During my early years I ate nothing but the best of foods, not necessarily rich, but whole and natural. We had little as far as material possessions, but we did eat well. Daddy always said, "We are what we eat." The only recipes I have remembered from childhood are those I watched him cook as I sat on the drain board countertop in our tiny kitchen with its icebox and small gas stove.

When my father died, I was 11 years old. My mother then became a single working parent of two children. With borrowed money she opened up a small dress shop. I grew up behind my mother's shop in three tiny rooms.

After marrying my teenage sweetheart, Bob Barnes, I became a mother of five children under five years of age. I was only 21. Three of the children were my brother's. His wife had walked out the door abandoning them all, and he could not take care of them. The years that followed gave me experience in preparing thousands of meals. We developed a natural foods lifestyle. With balanced nutrition our family was healthy, and yet the food was always tasty. We are not health nuts. We do eat chocolate chip cookies and waffles with maple syrup occasionally. We even enjoy chips and dip.

God has given me a heart's desire to teach women to be makers of their homes (Titus 2:4,5). Sue and I will share with you our secrets of tasty, nutritious, low-cost meals you can prepare as busy women in a fast-food world. You'll have more time, energy, and health to do the things you've always wanted to do. You will be blessed as you survive in a busy world with *More Hours In Your Day*. We will answer questions on eating out: where to go and what to order. We have prepared three dinner menus with recipe selections to get you started with the Eating Better Lifestyle: a 35-Day Unlimited Menu Plan, a 20-Day No Meat Plan, and a 20-Day No Dairy, No Egg Plan. Our recipes have passed the taste test of family and friends, receiving many compliments, too. They will add to your joy of cooking.

2

Sue's Story

I've always been interested in food preparation. My first serious venture was in high school home economics when I selected two weeks of planning and preparing family dinners as my special project. Not long after this, I was invited to plan and supervise the food service at a church retreat. Pursuing this interest, I enrolled in a university home economics program. In my freshman year I became a Christian through a dorm Bible study. It took me many years to understand, however, that what I learned through academic training too often ignored the values God had created in food.

Armed with a teaching credential, I taught two years of junior high and high school home economics. Meal planning centered on the Basic Four food groups. Appetite interest was enhanced by variety in color, tastes, textures, and temperatures. It was all based upon the use of white flour, white sugar, hydrogenated fats, meat as the main dish, and pre-packaged and canned foods. In addition to teaching and feeding my growing family, I was asked to manage the food service for many camps and retreats. That included seven beautiful summers at Campus by the Sea on Catalina Island where I received invaluable experience serving the American Diet to varying tastes of all ages in a facility without electricity or adequate refrigeration.

My awareness of the nutritional value of food began when I was pregnant with our fourth child. Inspired by Adele Davis' *Let's Have Healthy Children*, I managed to break the bottle barrier and nurse little Stephen for nine months. However, when he was a year old, he began to contract a series of sniffles and colds that sent us to the doctor. There I was supplied with antibiotics which I faithfully administered for ten full prescribed days on each occurrence. The runny nose

14

didn't stop. I began to question, "Didn't God create Stephen's body with an immune system that could fight off infection and disease?" I decided to stop running to the doctor for every little sniffle. Eventually my son's immune system took care of the problem. That gave me more incentive to find ways to help my family prevent and fight illness as the first preventive measure and make antibiotics and drugs the second measure.

In my research I discovered that some great gaps exist in the world between those who have little to eat and those who have an abundance. The irony is that both are hungry. The hunger of the first group is for a satisfied stomach. The unknown hunger of the second group (including myself and everyone else eating the American Diet) is for the nutritional values that technology has removed from the whole food sources. Reading Frances Moore Lappe's *Diet for a Small Planet*, I determined to do something about the world hunger problem. I read about how much grain it took to feed cattle so that affluent societies could enjoy a meat-centered diet. I tried some of the alternative meatless recipes on my family without success. My husband, Rich, was a meat-and-potatoes man, and even at age two our Stephen was a meat lover! The other children didn't get excited about tasteless bean-and-grain casseroles, either.

One day as I stood at my kitchen sink, I prayed, "Lord, is my interest in world hunger and nutrition wrong? Should I just forget about it?" In my mind a quiet, small voice prompted, "No, you are on the right track, but your timing is off, and your attitude is wrong. Trust Me, keep on researching and learning. Allow Me to change your attitude and give your husband and children receptivity to this new venture." I set aside my meatless meal experiments.

Soon a traumatic event changed the course of our lives. As our three-year-old Stephen was playing on the front lawn with his two older sisters, a drunken teenaged driver proceeded slowly down our street and struck our utility trailer and car. The trailer slammed over the curb and hit Stephen in the head as the driver continued down the street. While my husband breathed air into Stephen's limp, bleeding form, all I could pray was, "Jesus, help!"

Indeed, God does minister to our loss and grief through His miraculous gift of grace, love, and comfort. After a grave-side service, we shared a meal with close friends and family. One dear friend shared a passage of Scripture that was to become a cornerstone for our ministry. Isaiah 58:6-12 speaks of "spending yourselves on behalf of the hungry." Often during the ten years that have passed, my husband and I have returned to study that passage to remind ourselves of God's purpose and direction as we research, publish, and teach about food.

Within a few days one caring Christian neighbor sent a note expressing her concern. Encouraged, I visited her and shared our experience of God's comfort in our sorrow. She invited me to share my story with her Friday morning Bible study group which met at Emilie Barnes' home.

Several months later, Emilie Barnes and Florence Littauer held a seminar on how to be a godly woman in the home. Emilie included a ten-minute talk about nutrition. When she mashed a loaf of fluffy white bread into a mangled mass I was impressed. She didn't just stop with the squeeze. Pricking the ballooning plastic bread bag, she exploded it. It was evident that the number-one ingredient in that loaf of bread was air and what was left was at best calories with only a fraction of the original nutrients. Emilie dramatized what I was already beginning to discover about food. In fact, I had already purchased a bread kneader and flour mill and was preparing whole wheat breads, cinnamon rolls, and pizza for my family. My children and husband loved them! That was God's way of bringing change to my family. That day my dream to minister to women in the area of food and nutrition was born.

I began to read all of the books and articles on food preparation and nutrition that I could find. Rich, too, became interested. In fact, he took some tests and found out that he was actually a borderline diabetic! This unexpected revelation launched us into an even more serious investigation of how to change family food patterns. It seemed incredible that I hadn't learned these things during five years of home economics courses.

I began to read labels. My daughter Karen and I scoured the cupboards for all the questionable packaged foods, put them in a corner cupboard, and tied a string around the handles. We put ourselves to the test. If we could survive two weeks without them, perhaps we could do so for life. We did and we still do.

I learned how to prepare foods more complete in nutritional value. I learned about the values of fresh fruits and vegetables over canned, and how to fix a dinner without meat. Inevitably other people began to ask about the changes my family was making in food choices. As I began to share my whole grain breads, friends asked for the recipes. Informal kitchen sessions grew into demonstration classes. A few handout recipes expanded into two editions of *Natural Foods For All Occasions*, a recipe newsletter, the *Eating Better Cookbooks*, and a cooking demonstration video, "Eating Better with Sue."

Our family experienced positive results. My husband's prediabetic condition was quickly corrected. He lost excess weight and gained back his livable and loving disposition. His energy began to return. Dreams and goals supplanted depression. My son's frequent headaches and earaches diminished. Frequent visits to the doctor virtually ceased for all of us.

We realize that every aspect of our lives affects health and that nutritional change is not a guarantee of optimum health. Whatever the results, our desire is to reflect God's life-giving purpose for food in what we do with it. We have no intention of reverting back to the American Diet. We are committed because we believe that God has designed a life-giving nutritional plan for our benefit.

In addition to nutritional research, Rich and I began to investigate what the Bible had to say about food. With a concordance we checked out every reference we could find in the Bible about food or applicable to food. We found an incredible wealth of biblical principles, although not many recipes or menus. God knew what He was doing when He designed bodies and then created food for them. Our appreciation of Him as Creator and Provider expanded.

Every member of my family has not only benefited from the change but has also learned how to prepare wholesome foods. My son, Dan, has specialized in bread baking and served as a part-time cook in a college whole foods cafeteria. Karen, my older daughter, loves international cookery, is an excellent soup maker, and arranges beautiful fresh salads. Sharon, the youngest, is a real organizer in putting a whole meal together and serving it attractively, plus she bakes whole grain cookies and healthy desserts. Their future spouses and children, I believe, will receive special blessings through what they have learned. These skills, unfortunately, have been lost to the current generation. That is why my husband and I have committed ourselves to teaching others how to make the transition to eating better.

I appreciate the ideas that Emilie's smashed loaf of bread sparked. This demonstration helped me believe that it was possible to lead people from imitations to real God-given, life-producing food. With that same faith I believe that we can take charge of our lives—the way we eat, work, play, rest, minister to others, and worship.

3

Setting the Scene

> In the beginning God created the heavens and the earth. . . .God saw all that he had made, and it was very good.
>
> Genesis 1:1,31

This book has been written for one simple reason: We can eat better. Our families can eat better, too. Why? Because the typical twentieth-century American diet no longer adequately contains the nutritional value that God originally created in food. Current medical and scientific research has amply demonstrated that we are reaping the consequences in a host of daily health problems, degenerative diseases, and untimely deaths.

This should come as no surprise. Whenever mankind alters or ignores God's resources for life and health, tragic consequences follow. What a dishonor to Him who intended food to do good and not evil to mankind! He intended that the food He made for us would, instead, reap the benefits of health and well-being. It is that simple.

Yet we cannot promise you sensational health transformations. We cannot promise that you will lose 50 pounds, never get colds again, or never get cancer, heart disease, or diabetes. We cannot promise you that your energy will automatically soar. These and many other health benefits can and will happen to many people. Better nutrition will help each one of us where better nutrition is what our health needs. But since our health depends upon a whole complex of genetic, environmental, relational, and habitual lifestyle conditions, the benefits of eating better will vary widely. Nevertheless, nutrition does make a difference in the quality of our lives. And since God created food to be the vehicle of that nutrition, we honor Him when we pay attention to and utilize food's nutritional quality. We dishonor Him when we ignore good nutrition.

We believe that you will find this book unique in several ways. We do not expect our readers to treat the nutritional importance of food in an isolated or rigid way. Food means more than nutrition. It means family fellowship and celebration. It means security and comfort. It means cultural identity. It means giving, receiving, and sharing love. It is unrealistic to strive for better eating for nutrition's sake if these values that we place upon food are ignored, overlooked, or sacrificed. Therefore, we have approached this subject of eating better in the broader context of the role that food plays in our lives.

For example, the American dietary pattern is part of our cultural inheritance and is thus not easily abandoned for a strange diet, no matter how nutritional it may be. Hamburgers, spaghetti, pizza, and meat and potatoes are still in, but we can improve the nutritional quality through better choices of ingredients.

Many books attempt to achieve the ultimate in nutritional purity so that the many dos and don'ts lead to restriction rather than freedom. This leads to discouragement and failure. We want to introduce you to a wide range of choices you can enjoy with food of greater nutritional quality. We admit that we don't know everything there is to know about nutrition. Nobody does. There is controversy on many points. Therefore, we encourage you to make basic changes that have been well-established by scientific research. Then consider the range of choices we offer about the controversial issues. We will present you with these options rather than merely give you our own views as if they were the last word on the subject.

We do not pretend that the lifestyle change to eating better is simple. It is not. If you are to make lasting and permanent changes, you will need to make choices that will work well within the framework of your own circumstances. It will require commitment and perseverance to overcome obstacles. Some of these barriers are fears that can be allayed through better understanding. These are 1) How much time is required to focus on eating better? 2) How does it affect the food budget? 3) How is it all going to taste? Will the family like it? and 4) Where can the food resources be purchased? Other concerns are how to get started, how to help your family change, and how to choose better food when eating out.

Most women want practical help. This translates into where to buy the food, what to buy, and what recipes and menus to use. All the nutritional information in the world will not help if you do not have these resources. In Part 6 you will find dinner menu plans, the recipes to prepare them, and the help you need to buy the ingredients. If you are ready to start, don't wait to read all the nutrition and biblical background sections. Read Parts 2 and 3, Our Cultural Heritage and Coping With Change, for perspective and encouragement. Then you can treat Parts 4 and 5, the background sections, as a small encyclopedia if you wish. Look up the answers to your questions as they arise while you are choosing and preparing the recipes and menus.

God has set before us both life and death, and He calls us to choose life. Therefore, He will assist you in every way that you need to overcome obstacles to eating better. Every step you take will count for life. Look at your progress and be thankful for that, rather focusing on what still hasn't been done. God loves you infinitely and is willing to honor your commitment. Get organized and start moving. Do it with prayer. Your health and the health of your family is important to God. He desires to use you in our needy world to bring glory and honor to His name. To do that you need all the health and strength and vigor you can acquire.

That brings us to our final perspective in this book. It is biblically based. The health food movement has been primarily associated with the New Age Movement bringing in Eastern, Hinduistic philosophies. We will say more about this in later chapters. Here we want to note that when we see nutrition books that are associated with this philosophy of life on the shelves of Christian bookstores, we believe a confrontive biblical approach is needed.

There is much confusion in many believers' minds about the relationship of body and spirit. Few people recognize that the problem of eating better is an issue of spiritual conflict. Here are some reasons why we know this to be true. Physical food was God's first gift to mankind. He involved food's use in His test of man's obedience. Satan used food as an enticement for man's rebellion against Him. The Israelites' rebellion against God in the wilderness concerned food. Jesus' first temptation by the devil in the wilderness was a food temptation. The first contention that arose in the early church was over a matter of food distribution. The expression of the most important spiritual truth of all time—that Jesus Christ died on the cross for sins—is represented by the food symbols of bread and wine, established by Jesus Christ Himself.

Satan is a thief who steals, kills, and destroys. If he can do it through nutritionally poor food, which he is doing on a grand scale, he will. If he can do it by associating anti-Christian philosophies with good food, he will do that, too. We need to prayerfully ask God for discernment.

The following chapters introduce you to a broad variety of nutritional and practical food issues, many of which we have mentioned in this chapter. Where we have found other books to be good resources on a particular topic we have named those at appropriate places. These references have then been listed together on a Recommended Reading list in the Appendix. We encourage you to get involved right away in the action in Part 6 with recipes and menus as you read this book.

4

What Are the Benefits?

> . . . he himself gives all men life and breath and everything else. . . . For in him we live and move and have our being.
>
> Acts 17:25,28

The measure of health one has is dependent upon a healthy system of digestion and elimination. All the other processes of the body are strengthened by it, such as the immune, circulatory, or lymphatic systems, for example. We fail to appreciate these benefits fully because we cannot see them happening. But we can appreciate the results in our daily lives. Eating a healthy balance of life-giving food will contribute to benefits that we all desire:

—Better weight control
—More youthful appearance—healthier skin, hair, eyes
—More energy
—Greater mental alertness
—More stable emotions
—Freedom from common digestive discomforts
—Increased resistance to illness
—Increased resistance to degenerative diseases
—Faster and more complete healing of injuries
—Slower aging—longer life

These benefits will also result in:

—Less money needed for medical bills
—Less time spent in bed, in doctors' offices, in hospitals
—More freedom to enjoy and love family and friends
—More freedom for ministry and service to God

5

Grandpa Ate Everything and Lived to 92!

> He makes grass grow for the cattle, and plants for man to cultivate—bringing forth food from the earth: wine that gladdens the heart of man, oil to make his face shine, and bread that sustains his heart.
>
> Psalm 104:14,15

Someone's hail-and-hearty grandpa always manages to have enjoyed eating what he liked on his journey to a ripe old age! If he could do it, why can't I? How did grandpa manage? To answer that we must hearken back to grandpa's childhood on the family farm.

Grandpa was a hardworking young man from the time he could collect the daily egg quota. No time for lying down on the job. The cows needed milking, the garden needed weeding, the crops needed harvesting. School and studies took up the evening hours. There were special occasions, though, for socializing, fun, and feasting. These were big events and included the usual broad spread of farm-fresh beef, pork, chicken, fresh vegetables, homemade gravy, fresh hot rolls with lots of churned butter, milk, and hot apple, cherry, and pumpkin pies with homemade ice cream. In fact, everyday meals were a simplified version of such feasts as these, calculated to satisfy the appetites of farmers who worked from dawn till dusk.

In grandpa's day the air in the country was fresh, clear, and unpolluted. The water from the creek was pure. Pesticides and herbicides were unheard of. Farm-fresh produce was organic and uncontaminated. Seasonal produce brought ripe from vine and tree to the dining table was a way of life. The foods you didn't grow on your own, you often did not have to eat. Available meats and poultry were lean and free of antibiotics and growth stimulants. Fish came from unpolluted streams and rivers. Although meats, fish, and poultry were available, if grandpa lived at the turn of the century, he was probably eating more of his protein in beans, grains, and vegetables.

There were lean times, too. The depression years provided an especially prolonged time of frugal fare. Hearty eating was not always one long and unending feast from birth to the grave. Lean times may well have provided many digestive systems with a needed respite from more sumptuous seasons. The daily struggles against the caprice of the elements provided experiences that firmed up resolve and fortitude. Family values, social and moral standards, and the work ethic were all more clearly delineated, understood, and lived by. All of these living patterns contributed to grandpa's hail-and-hearty condition.

Alas! Grandpa's world is no longer our world. In fact, not too many grandpas or favorite old uncles are living to a ripe old age anymore, at least not without the typical health traumas of cancers, heart attacks, diabetes, and Alzheimer's disease. What has happened? How has our world and food supply changed? What have we inherited?

6

Whatever Happened to the Basic Four?

> I brought you into a fertile land to eat its fruit and rich produce. But you came and defiled my land and made my inheritance detestable.
>
> Jeremiah 2:7

Grandpa was little concerned with the nutrition in his food. He just ate and lived or ate and got sick, most often from something other than what was lacking in his food. His food may not have been perfect, but there were many other contributions to health in his life to compensate for what was lacking. Grandpa got what nutrients he could because much of what he needed still remained intact in his food. Although he certainly was consuming some white flour and white sugar in a variety of recipes, his generation was not yet reaping the full effect of this devitalization. Fresh and lean farm products also helped to make up for the lack. Practically everything he ate was freshly prepared in the home kitchen. Almost all of the young women in his day learned how to cook from basic foods.

The first vitamin, vitamin B_2, was not discovered until 1886 by Casimir Funk. A full quarter of our twentieth century was gone before Albert Szent-Gyorgyi discovered vitamin C. Gyorgyi expressed appropriate appreciation. "Vitamins . . . will help us to reduce human suffering to an extent which the most fantastic mind would fail to imagine."[1] Of course, the Creator imagined it from the beginning and knew all along what He had put into food for our benefit. The discoveries of nutritional research have mushroomed since Gyorgyi's discovery.

As new information about food was learned, new tools for educating the American population were developed. The

Basic Seven food groups were classified as a practical guideline to planning nutritious meals. Later, the Basic Seven was simplified to the Basic Four food groups. Specific size and number of servings were designated for each food group. The plan was easy to follow because it focused on groups of actual foods that could be harvested, stored, prepared, and tasted, rather than on nutrients hidden in the foods.

The Basic Four plan was ideal in a rural economy. The food groups very simply reflected farm fare—meats, fish, poultry, eggs, beans; dairy products; fruits and vegetables; and breads and cereals.

Another food revolution was about to occur. The advent of modern food technology ushered in supermarket shelves full of new food products of which white flour and white sugar of the previous century were only a forerunner. Most of these new products were and are different versions on the same theme—refined foods such as white flour and white sugar, stripped of major portions of fiber and nutrients, and dressed up with a wide variety of chemicals that never were part of the original food. Twinkies and Fruit Loops joined the home-baked white breads and pie crusts. Public consumption of these new products began to escalate. In addition, cattlemen were beginning to develop new ways to produce juicier and more tender meats. As the population was migrating to the cities, there was an increased need for fruits and vegetables preserved for those who didn't grow their own. An increasing variety of fruits and vegetables commercially canned in sugar syrups or with salt entered the market.

Unfortunately, most of these new food products fit neatly into the Basic Four food groups. One can eat the proper daily allotment of the Basic Four by having juicy beef filled with antibiotics and excessive fat, canned fruits in sugar syrup, salty canned vegetables, processed American cheese, chocolate ice cream, white toast, Fruit Loops, and Twinkies. Thousands upon thousands of food products developed since World War II make it not only possible, but a reality in most American households for people to get plenty to eat while eating relatively few basic whole foods. This is true even when the Basic Four food plan is followed.

It is apparent that a different food plan is needed to give adequate guidance for selecting nutritious foods and menus. The charts which follow describe the present American Diet and the Eating Better Lifestyle. The contrast between these two is then summarized. The menu plans with recipes in Part 6 reflect the guidelines of the Eating Better Lifestyle.

THE AMERICAN DIET

Percents (%) are percentages of calories.

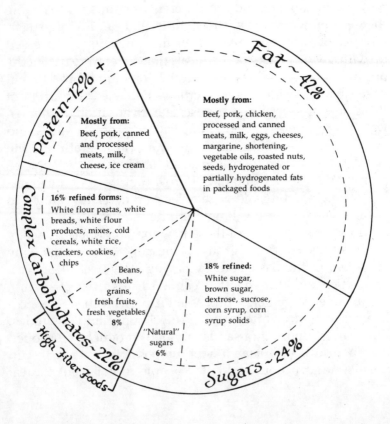

Fat ~42%

Mostly from:
Beef, pork, chicken, processed and canned meats, milk, eggs, cheeses, margarine, shortening, vegetable oils, roasted nuts, seeds, hydrogenated or partially hydrogenated fats in packaged foods

Protein-12% +

Mostly from:
Beef, pork, canned and processed meats, milk, cheese, ice cream

Complex Carbohydrates ~22%

16% refined forms:
White flour pastas, white breads, white flour products, mixes, cold cereals, white rice, crackers, cookies, chips

Beans, whole grains, fresh fruits, fresh vegetables 8%

High Fiber Foods

"Natural" sugars 6%

18% refined:
White sugar, brown sugar, dextrose, sucrose, corn syrup, corn syrup solids

Sugars ~24%

THE EATING BETTER LIFESTYLE

Percents (%) are percentages of calories.

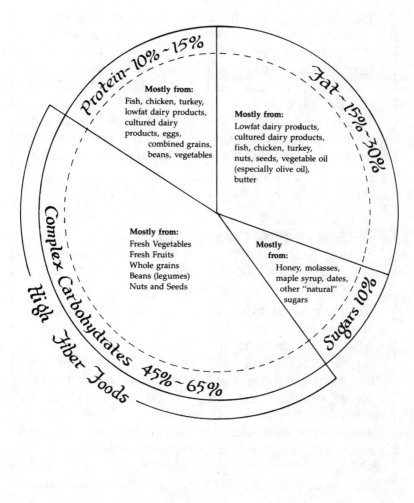

Protein-10%~15%

Mostly from:
Fish, chicken, turkey,
lowfat dairy products,
cultured dairy
products, eggs,
combined grains,
beans, vegetables

Fat~15%~30%

Mostly from:
Lowfat dairy products,
cultured dairy products,
fish, chicken, turkey,
nuts, seeds, vegetable oil
(especially olive oil),
butter

Mostly from:
Fresh Vegetables
Fresh Fruits
Whole grains
Beans (legumes)
Nuts and Seeds

Mostly
from:
Honey, molasses,
maple syrup, dates,
other "natural"
sugars

Sugars 10%

Complex Carbohydrates 45%~65%

High Fiber Foods

TAKING A LOOK AT THE DIFFERENCE

THE TYPICAL AMERICAN DIET

- High in Meat & Dairy Foods
- High in Refined Carbohydrates
- Low in Unrefined Carbohydates
- 10,000 mg. to 20,000 mg. sodium/day
- HIGH FAT—LOW FIBER

Deficient (or Devitalized): Refined carbohydrates are deficient in original fiber, vitamins, minerals, and unknown nutritional properties.

Unbalanced: Excessive refined sugars and starches, fats, meat and dairy protein, and sodium (10,000 to 20,000 milligrams per day).

Adulterated: A large portion of these foods contains many added chemicals suspect to human health—pesticide residues, preservatives, artificial colorings, and flavorings.

EATING BETTER LIFESTYLE

- Low in Meat & Dairy Foods
- Low in Refined Carbohydrates
- High in Unrefined Carbohydrates
- 1,100 mg. to 3,300 mg. sodium/day
- LOW FAT—HIGH FIBER

The menus and recipes on pp. 223-78 aim toward developing the Eating Better Lifestyle pattern.

More Complete Nutrient Supply: More whole (unrefined) complex carbohydrate foods contain more original fiber, vitamins, minerals, and unknown nutritional properties.

Better Balance: Less refined sugars and starches, fat, meat protein, and sodium (1,100 mg. to 3,300 mg. per day).

Less Adulterated: A large portion of these foods contains a significantly lower amount of chemicals suspect to human health.

7

God's Cornucopia of Whole Foods

> Then God said, "I give you every seed-bearing plant on the face of the whole earth and every tree that has fruit with seed in it. They will be yours for food. . . . Everything that lives and moves will be food for you. Just as I gave you the green plants, I now give you everything."
>
> Genesis 1:29; 9:3

When Sue was developing a whole foods quantity program for a college cafeteria, she requested some evaluations. One student responded, "Health food is not in the Bible." He included a series of Scriptures to prove the point! This evaluation reflected the idea that biblically there are no right foods to eat, especially not ones that you don't like!

We agree that there are many health-food products that don't taste very good, at least not to the American palate. That, however, is an evaluation of the recipes used, not of the basic food ingredients used in the products. Most health-food products do use basic food ingredients that are closer to the way God made them than typical American food fare. In this sense, health food most certainly is in the Bible. But our understanding and, indeed, our appreciation for basic whole foods will be enhanced if we can separate them from the man-produced recipes and menus they are used in. Making the basic whole foods tasty in recipes and menus is a separate issue and the subject of the next chapter.

Let's look at God's cornucopia of whole foods generally available to most Americans, either seasonally or year-round.

There are approximately:

10 *Whole Grains*—barley, brown rice, buckwheat, cornmeal, oats, millet, wheat, rye, triticale, amaranth

16 *Legumes* (dry beans and peas)—red, kidney, pinto, black-eyed, black, split pea, fava, navy, lima, mung, soy, garbanzo, lentils, great northern, peanuts, azuki

16 *Nuts and Seeds*—almonds, Brazil nuts, cashews, coconut, filberts, macadamia nuts, pecans, pine nuts, pistachio nuts, walnuts, pumpkin seeds, sunflower seeds, sesame seeds, caraway seeds, poppy seeds, alfalfa seeds

60 *Fresh Vegetables*

33 *Fresh Fruits*

7 *Dairy Products*—sweet milk, cream, butter, soft cheeses, hard cheeses, eggs, cultured milks

4 *Meats and Poultry*—beef, lamb, chicken, turkey

20 *Fish*

20 *Herbs and Spices*

1 *First-Choice Sweetener*—honey

Think for a moment, if you will, of the many ways in which these basic whole foods can be prepared and combined in recipes and menus. The exponential possibilities are staggering!

Is it not wonderful that God chose to give us such food variety to work with? He so easily could have provided us only with manna just as He did for the Israelites in the wilderness for 40 years. But it is evident that God loves variety and has lavishly displayed it in creation. It reflects the awesomeness of His glory and power. God's Word tells us that His

". . . invisible qualities—his eternal power and divine nature—have been clearly seen, being understood from what has been made. . . ." (Romans 1:20). Imagine it! We are called upon to recognize God's eternal power and divine nature from the food He has created! How is that possible if the foods we eat are so devitalized* and adulterated* that they are significant contributors to such things as cancers, heart disease, diabetes, overweight, and a host of other unhappy ills? The chart on pages 34-35 illustrates this. On the contrary, foods are meant to give life because they originated out of the invisible qualities of our life-giving God. If we, His children, are to reflect the character of our heavenly Father, then we too must seek to utilize food in a life-giving way. He has provided us with a wealth of life-giving whole foods in order to do that.

---

*Devitalized means that many of the life-giving nutrients have been processed out of the food. Adulterated means that chemicals not originally in the food have been added for preservation, coloring, and flavoring.

Whole Wheat: A Lesson in Nutritional Loss

Nutrients Available in Whole Wheat Flour	Nutrient Loss in All-Purpose White Flour[1]
Vitamins	
thiamine (B_1)*	77%
riboflavin (B_2)*	67%
niacin (B_3)*	81%
pyridoxine (B_6)	72%
choline (part of B-complex)	30%
folic acid (part of B-complex)	67%
pantothenic acid (part of B-complex)	50%
vitamin E	86%
Minerals	
chromium	40%
manganese	86%
selenium	16%
zinc	98%
iron*	75%
cobalt	89%
calcium	60%
sodium	78%
potassium	77%
magnesium	85%
phosphorus	91%
molybdenum	48%
copper	68%
Total average loss	70%

*These nutrients are added to "enriched" white flour in synthetic form, but are not restored in the original natural form.

Dietary Fiber   89%
   (1 cup whole wheat = 14.4
     grams)
   (1 cup white flour = 1.6
     grams)

Undiscovered nutrient value   unknown
of wheat germ and bran

Approximately 50% of the American Diet is refined carbohydrate. Most of it is in the form of these food items prepared from all-purpose white flour:

> noodles, spaghetti, macaroni, lasagna noodles, cake mixes, cookie mixes, pancake mixes, frozen waffles, breakfast cereals, sandwich breads, hot dog buns, hamburger buns, English muffins, flour tortillas, pita breads, bread mixes, prepackaged pasta mixes, pizza, crackers, cakes, cookies, donuts, croissants, sweet rolls, muffins, biscuit and roll mixes, dinner rolls

A good portion of refined carbohydrate also comes from white rice and degerminated cornmeal, white rice mixes, cornmeal mixes, corn tortillas, and corn chips devitalized in the same way as white flour.

8

The Recipe Box—Using God's Resources Imaginatively

Let us make man in our image, in our likeness, and let them rule over the fish of the sea and the birds of the air, over the livestock, over all the earth, and over all the creatures that move along the ground.

Genesis 1:26

Have you ever wondered why there are many listings of foods in the Bible but few, if any, recipes and menus? Obviously the creation of recipes, menus, and cookbooks is our privileged domain. More cookbooks are published and sold than any other subject category. The endless variety of recipes from family to family, region to region, and culture to culture reflects how well we imitate the Creator!

Now we have the opportunity to fulfill the divine design by choosing the best of God's whole food provisions and by handling those foods with care. The standard we've chosen for the recipes in this book comes from Deuteronomy 30:19,20:— "Now choose life, so that you and your children may live . . . For the LORD is your life, and he will give you many years in the land. . . ." It is our aim to constantly be alert to new food sources, new food preparation techniques, and food combinations in recipes and menus that maximize the life-giving benefits of God's wonderful provision.

At the same time we are aware that a brief encounter with "health foods" (foods that are "good" for you) has provided many with their first and decidedly last encounter. There are two reasons why. First, health food advocates have often forgotten that taste buds have no brains. That means that appetites are whetted by sensual responses, not by nutritional analyses. Secondly, health foods too often begin with the unfamiliar (e.g. macrobiotic or vegetarian) rather than with familiar foods.

Every cultural group has a distinct dietary pattern. While there is great diversity in the cultural backgrounds of Americans, there is an American pattern (witness the same menus served by restaurant chains from coast to coast and even overseas!) as opposed, say, to a Japanese or Mexican pattern. In the recipes and menus in this book we've chosen not to abandon all the American favorites, but to improve the quality of the familiar while introducing the new. The Minute Bran Muffin recipe that follows illustrates what a difference just improving the ingredients of a familiar recipe can make!

Taste and appetite are God-given just as the indispensable nutrients in food are God-given. The challenge to us is to create a variety of recipes and menus that offer both.

Two Ways to Use God's Whole Food Resources

Recipe: **MINUTE BRAN MUFFINS**		
Basic Ingredients	American Diet Choice	Eating Better Lifestyle Choice
Wheat bran	1½ cups bran cereal	1½ cups unprocessed
Flour	1½ cups all-purpose	1½ cups whole wheat
Sugar	1 cup brown sugar	⅓ cup honey
Fat	½ cup shortening	
Egg	1	1
Buttermilk	1 cup	1 cup
Soda	1¼ teaspoons	1¼ teaspoons
Salt	1¼ teaspoons	1 teaspoon
NUTRITION RESULTS Per Muffin		
Calories	284	145
Protein	5 grams	5 grams
Fat	11.6 grams	1.7 grams
% of Calories in fat	37%	10%
Vitamins and Minerals	70% less in flour*	70% more in flour*
Dietary Fiber	4.3 grams	6 grams
Sugar	6.3 teaspoons	1.3 teaspoons
Sodium	489 milligrams	369 milligrams
Cost	$.11	$.06

---

*See "total average loss," p. 34.

MINUTE BRAN MUFFINS*   10 to 12 Large

These go with everything! Serve warm or cold.

Preheat oven at 350°. Grease muffin pan or line with muffin papers.

Cover with warm water and let stand 5 to 10 minutes:
½ cup raisins (optional)

Blend together and let stand for 5 minutes:
½ cup boiling water
1½ cups unprocessed wheat bran (Miller's)

Blend together thoroughly in order given with wire whisk:
1 egg
¼ to ⅓ cup honey
1 cup buttermilk or sour milk
bran mixture

Blend dry ingredients together in separate bowl:
1½ cups whole wheat or whole wheat pastry flour
1¼ teaspoons soda
1 teaspoon salt
½ cup walnuts, chopped (optional)

Blend drained raisins, then dry ingredients into liquid ingredients just until mixed. Do not overmix!

Bake 20 to 25 minutes.
Cool 5 to 10 minutes before removing from pan.

1 muffin (10 per recipe)—raisins/walnuts not included:

145 calories, 4.5 grams protein, 32 grams carbohydrate, 1.5 grams fat (11% of calories), 6 grams dietary fiber

---

* This recipe also included in recipe section, p. 270.

9

Eating Better Lifestyle Alternatives

> The man who eats everything must not look down on him who does not, and the man who does not eat everything must not condemn the man who does, for God has accepted him.
>
> Romans 14:3

Romans 14 teaches that there is more than one way to eat and that people ought not to judge one another for choosing different ways. Romans 14 does not teach that it doesn't matter what we eat. There are several criteria for making proper choices of food in Romans 14. For example Romans 14:5 says that "Each one should be fully convinced in his own mind." That guideline suggests that some intelligent forethought should be given to choices of food. Romans 14:23 teaches that what we eat should be a matter of faith. Mature Christian faith should be based on facts that reflect God's character and purpose rather than merely upon one's cultural tradition or personal tastes.

At this time there is much new and conflicting teaching about what is the most healthy way to eat. Nutrition certainly falls in the category of "disputable matters" (Romans 14:1). We need to be patient with both the situation and with others who choose different plans of eating. We believe there is adequate scriptural and scientific grounds for encouraging a change to the Eating Better Lifestyle, and also for defining what that lifestyle is. But there are several alternative dietary patterns that fit the Eating Better Lifestyle framework. These include: 1) The Unlimited Plan; 2) The Lacto-Vegetarian Plan; 3) The Vegan Vegetarian Plan; 4) The No Dairy-No Egg Plan; 5) The Limited Food Combination Plan; 6) The Low Sodium

Plan; 7) The Extra Low Fat Plan; and 8) The Therapeutic Diet Plan. We do not claim that these are the only Eating Better Lifestyle diet plans but they are the ones that have drawn the broadest attention among Americans, and they are the ones that we want to define in this book.

These alternatives may be briefly described as follows:

1) *The Unlimited Plan* does not exclude any major food groups. Meats, dairy products, fruits, vegetables, grains, beans, nuts, seeds, and natural sugars are all included. We have included a 35-Day Planned Menu in Part 6 using this plan.

2) *The Lacto-Vegetarian Plan* includes dairy products and sometimes eggs, and excludes meat, fish, and poultry. Part 6 includes a 20-Day Planned Dinner Menu excluding meats.

3) *The Vegan Vegetarian Plan* includes plant foods only—no eggs, no dairy products, no meat, fish, or poultry. Care must be taken when following the vegan diet to get enough calcium and vitamin B_{12}. The best plant sources of calcium are broccoli and dark leafy green vegetables. B_{12} can be supplied through seaweed or supplements. Several of our recipes are suitable for the vegan menu.

4) *The No-Dairy, No-Egg Plan* includes meats, fish, and poultry but excludes eggs and dairy products. Part 6 includes a 20-Day No-Dairy, No-Egg Dinner Menu Plan.

5) *The Limited Food Combinations Plan* follows several rules of combining foods but in essence they are: a) Eat fruits alone; b) Eat starchy carbohydrates with vegetables; c) Eat proteins with vegetables. Other combinations are not recommended. Several of the recipes in Part 6 are suitable for this plan.

6) *The Low Sodium Plan* limits sodium intake to 500 milligrams per day. To maintain this level, salt additions must be omitted from food. The Recommended Daily Allowance of sodium is 1,100 to 3,300 milligrams. The menus in Part 6 are within the RDA limit. Salt may be omitted from the recipes.

7) *The Extra Low Fat Plan* limits fat intake to 12%-17% of calories. Menus in Part 6 are within the USDA recommended limit of 30% or less calories of fat. Many of our recipes are in

the 12%-17% range.

8) *The Therapeutic Diet Plan* is any diet plan that is more or less tailor-made for an individual with specific health problems. Most of the recipes in Part 6 are easily adaptable for use in therapeutic diets.

It is our desire to make the Eating Better Lifestyle as flexible and useful to as many needs, tastes, interests, and nutritional convictions that we can. It is a very flexible eating lifestyle. Also, you may be assured that each one of these alternatives, with good planning, will provide adequate nutrition. Restrictions aside, they are all superior in health benefits to the American Diet.

10

First Things First

Have I not commanded you? Be strong and coura-
geous. Do not be terrified; do not be discouraged,
for the LORD your God will be with you wherever
you go.

Joshua 1:9

When the Israelites had crossed the Red Sea, Moses sent 12
men into Canaan to survey the land and bring back some of its
abundant fresh produce. Only two of the men, Joshua and
Caleb, returned with the optimistic report that they could
conquer the land. The remaining ten men saw only the strong
fortified cities filled with powerful people (Numbers 13). The
difference between their fear and Joshua's and Caleb's confidence was the faith that God had already promised to give
them the land. Would God give such a promise without
providing His presence and strength to fulfill it?

The fear of changing our eating lifestyle is a legitimate
one considering that almost everything needs to be totally
overhauled! So much is involved—the taste preferences of
everyone we feed, finding new shopping resources, developing new food preparation skills, new menu planning, new
food storage methods, new food budgeting, and new recipes.

God commanded Joshua to be strong and unafraid because
his task was God-given. The first step in making the Eating
Better Lifestyle change is commitment to the Lord for "It is
the Lord Christ you are serving" (Colossians 3:24).

Next, develop the Eating Better Lifestyle one step at a time.
Don't try to do everything at once. Note how Moses sent the
men to survey the land before launching campaigns to conquer it (Numbers 13). Use the whys and how-tos of this book
to plan your own strategy and time schedule. Don't judge

your progress by someone else's standard. Concentrate on making the basic changes first.

The menus, recipes, suggestions for improving your own favorite recipes, and guidelines for dining out in Part 6 reflect the following basic changes:

> *more fiber*: include more whole grains, dry beans, fresh fruits, and fresh vegetables
>
> *more vitamins and minerals*: same as above
>
> *less fat*: reduce red meats, reduce use of vegetable oils, margarine, butter, and shortening in cooking and in packaged foods; add more fiber as above; use more of the lowfat dairy products and cheeses
>
> *less refined sugar*: cut amount by half—use honey in place of sugar; omit canned and packaged foods with sugar
>
> *less sodium*: leave salt off the table; reduce canned and packaged food items that contain salt; do not add salt to vegetables
>
> *controlled calories*: all of the above will contribute wonderfully—without counting!

Leave detailed refinements for later when you have begun to feel more comfortable with the Eating Better Lifestyle. For example, arrowroot powder is more nutritious than cornstarch, but it is a minor ingredient in comparison to white flour versus whole grain flour. For another example, choosing organically grown produce* has merit, but choosing more fresh fruits and vegetables of any kind is more important. The point is, major on the majors.

---

*See definition, p. 143.

11

Overcoming the Four Fears

If you falter in times of trouble, how small is your strength! Proverbs 24:10

I can do everything through him who gives me strength. Philippians 4:13

People considering the Eating Better Lifestyle face four fears: 1) "I am afraid it won't taste good"; 2) "I am afraid it will take too much time"; 3) "I am afraid it will cost too much"; and 4) "I am afraid it will be too difficult to find the ingredients."

What About Taste?

Appealing taste is the single most important reason why we choose to eat what we do. People often give other excuses for not changing their eating patterns when the real reason is fear of unfamiliar taste. Sue's technically oriented friend, Bob, a California Institute of Technology graduate, thought that he needed all the nutrient data to prove the value of whole foods first. That was true until he ate our four-grain pancakes! He loved them. It was the satisfaction of that taste which motivated him to change his eating habits.

The frequent criticism of health food is that it does not taste good. We agree. Why? One reason is that too many health enthusiasts become too restrictive in their choices of ingredients and recipes. Some leave all the salt and all the fat out of recipes. The result is bland and blah food. It takes real skill to find other seasonings to compensate. Another problem is that many health food advocates expect people to adopt a menu and recipe pattern that is not American—no more hamburgers, no more pizza, no more meat and potatoes. Our recipes are certainly not all hamburgers and pizza, but they retain the familiar American tastes. Katherine's comment reflects a typical response: "My family has enjoyed the food I've cooked from your books. I feel a peaceful balance in our eating and don't feel so frustrated in my attempts to provide good nutrition."

We'd like to share our secret of how to develop good-tasting recipes. Here are some simple guidelines. First, start with recipes and menus familiar to your family's tastes but improve the nutritional quality of some of the ingredients. For example, instead of cutting hamburgers out of the menu, use meat that is lower in fat such as ground turkey. Then put it on whole wheat hamburger buns instead of white bread buns. Check out Part 6 for more ideas on this. Second, read the salt and fat chapters to see why you don't have to cut all the salt and fat out of recipes. Third, change those things first that your tastes can handle. So tofu and brown rice don't appeal to you now—try whole wheat spaghetti instead. If you aren't ready for whole wheat flour, try half whole wheat and half white flour.

Finally, be patient with yourself and those you serve. Remember that the objective is to win the war, not just a little skirmish. Experiment with new recipes. Don't expect everyone to like everything. It may take two years before you hear the words that one young mother finally heard from her once-skeptical husband, "Dear, I want you to try every recipe in that book!"

God has created enough variety for you to select what appeals to your family. Trust the One who created taste buds for His whole foods to give you skill and wisdom in choosing and timing your presentations of new dishes.

The white flour and brown sugar cinnamon rolls that I (Sue) once baked for summer campers on Catalina Island were the highlight of each week's breakfasts. Later after I learned to bake cinnamon rolls with honey and whole wheat flour for my family, we returned to camp. We discovered that the white flour, refined sugary cinnamon rolls lacked the satiating satisfaction we had learned to enjoy in the whole-grain-and-honey version, and we realized then that our taste buds could, indeed, adapt to enjoy the flavors and textures of food for which they were created.

We use a family rating scale to evaluate the taste of new recipes (p. 55). It can be a real help in assisting the transition. To assure your success we've put taste as the first priority in selecting the recipes and menus in Part 6.

What About Time?

> There is a time for everything, and a season for every activity under heaven.
>
> Ecclesiastes 3:1

Fast-food outlets, TV dinners, prepackaged foods, and the microwave oven are rapidly producing a generation of noncooks. Lack of time has become a real obstacle to quality home food preparation because there are so many alternatives to cooking. Does developing the Eating Better Lifestyle now mean that we must spend hours slaving in our kitchens? No!

No one has been given more than 24 hours for each day. The secret is not to get more time. It is to manage our time. It takes only a little time to plan the saving of much time. This is the purpose of Emilie's More Hours In My Day Seminars. During the initial period of transition, the Eating Better Lifestyle requires careful planning. That is why we have included a section in Part 6 on how to do it. In addition, more help is available beyond what we have covered in this book (p. 287).

Save the more complex recipes for later. Start with supermarket ingredients that require very simple preparation such as Brown Rice (p. 226) or Lentil Rice Casserole (p. 228). Many prepackaged whole food items of nutritional quality are now available. Just remember to read the label! For example, whole grain breads and pastas are now on many supermarket shelves. You will find more wholesome frozen entrées too.

Your freezer can become a real timesaver in reducing frequent trips to the market. Even though Sue has access to three supermarkets within ¾ mile of her home, her favorite multigrain bread (ten grains plus two legumes) comes from a store 20 miles away. When she's on business trips she stops and purchases 10 to 12 loaves at a time to put in the freezer.

Baking, especially yeast breads, is one of the more complex food tasks. Marvelous machines now will perform much of the time-consuming labor for you. A flour mill makes the preparation of fresh whole grain quick breads almost as easy as opening a packaged mix, and a bread kneader/food processor takes the kneading work out of yeast bread preparation. It is also easier to buy and store the grains than the flours.

You will discover that some foods such as unpeeled potatoes actually take less time than the less nutritious peeled potatoes. Most fresh fruit can be eaten as is while canned fruit requires a can opener.

Don't forget to include your children in food preparation. If they fix it, they will eat it. Little hands may be messy now, but they can become timesavers for you later when they plan the menus, do the shopping, and prepare some of the meals (as our children in their teens have done). As they become independent young adults, they will leave your home with valuable survival skills.

Taking time to plan the family food strategy is part of our God-given role. Food manufacturers and merchandizers would like to get us to pay them to do it for us. Part of their persuasive tactic is to convince us that unpaid, unrecognized service is also unworthy. Not so with Jesus. For example, in Luke 8:2,3 a group of women (much better off financially) followed Jesus and His disciples and provided for their physical needs. This freed Jesus to give His time to preaching and healing. In Acts 6:1-7 the apostles appointed men with the highest spiritual qualifications for the service of food distribution: "We will turn this responsibility over to them and will give our attention to prayer and the ministry of the word" (verses 3,4). Not only is providing food a necessary task, it is worthy of godly attention by some in order to free others to carry out the work God has given them to do.

What About Cost?

> Why spend money on what is not bread, and your labor on what does not satisfy? Listen, listen to me, and eat what is good, and your soul will delight in the richest of fare.
>
> Isaiah 55:2

Losing one's health is a costly ordeal. The average yearly medical cost per person in America is now $1,500 per year. In addition to medical costs, the cost of days of work lost through illness runs in the millions. In fact, some corporations have begun fitness programs for employees. These programs are proving to be less costly than the employee days of work lost. These businesses are learning that preventive measures to maintain health are an economic benefit.

Good nutrition is an economical preventive health-care measure. Eating nutritionally inferior food saves neither money nor life. Such foods fill the stomach but fail to satisfy the real nutrient needs of the body. Jamie discovered this with her son, Tim. Tim missed 47 days of school and spent seven-and-a-half days in the hospital in the second and third grade. His medical costs were over $1,000 for one year. Jamie's family began the Eating Better Lifestyle as Tim entered the fourth grade. In the three years that followed Tim missed five days of school and there were no medical expenses!

The USDA issues quarterly reports of changes in individual and family food costs for eating at home. They are divided into four categories: thrifty, low budget, moderate budget, and liberal. We should note, however, that the amount spent does not reflect the difference between a poor diet or a good diet.

Where we eat makes a great difference as to what food costs. By 1983 Americans were eating 42% of their meals in restaurants. In 1984 Americans spent $1,800 per person in fast-food restaurants,[1] an average of almost $5.00 per day, higher than the liberal budget food plan of eating at home in 1986. Usually we will find enough money to buy what we consider important. Certainly, we can trust our God to give us the wisdom to spend wisely for good nutrition what money we do have for food.

While some Eating Better Lifestyle foods are more costly item for item, the overall cost may be less expensive. Note the cost, for example of the Minute Bran Muffins (p. 38). Our muffins are less expensive than the typical American muffins. While the whole wheat flour and the honey are more expensive ingredients than white flour and white sugar, the unprocessed bran is less expensive than bran cereal, and the shortening, a costly ingredient, is not used in the more nutritious muffins.

We also significantly shift the expense of the food bill when we purchase smaller amounts of high fat, high protein foods such as meats and dairy products. This gives us more dollars to spend on some of the more nutritious food items such as whole grains and fresh vegetables. These can be combined in delicious recipes with herbs for flavoring and a little meat added. The end result is a menu that is less costly than the menu using a prepacked refined food item and a larger meat serving.

When considering the real expense of food, we must think in terms of value received for dollars spent. Refined pre-packaged foods will always cost more than basic food staples. You will always pay for the labor of pre-prepared food, its fancy packaging to attract your attention, and the advertising to encourage you to buy it. Basic food staples such as grains, dry beans, fresh fruits, and vegetables get little advertising promotion, are not generally put into fancy packaging, and require little pre-preparation. More of your food dollar is therefore being spent on the nutritional value.

There are many ways to economize the food budget without sacrificing nutritional value. Here are several. Even if you choose to do only one or two of them you will realize a significant savings:

—Bake whole grain breads rather than buy them.
—Grow, rather than buy, sprouts.
—Grow as much as you can in your own garden—feed the soil with your food scraps for a rich growing medium instead of feeding them to the disposal or garbage can. Have a covered container conveniently located in the kitchen in which to put your food scraps—empty it once a day into your outdoor compost heap.
—Take advantage of in-season fruits and vegetables.
—Take advantage of sales on nutritious basic food items.
—Reduce the number of desserts in your menu.
—Participate in a food co-op.
—Utilize leftovers wisely.
—Plan your menus.
—Shop only from a planned grocery list.
—Minimize your shopping trips.
—Purchase nonperishable food items or items that keep well in the freezer in quantity or economy sizes (a freezer is a wise economy investment, especially for the single person who uses smaller amounts of many perishable items).
—Limit visits to restaurants and fast-food outlets. Share meals.
—Don't buy every "health food" alternative for every "junk food" available (such as cookies, candy, etc.).
—Use meats more frequently in small amounts as a supplement to dinner menus rather than the main food item.
—Have several "meatless" meals during the week.
—Develop the habit of drinking more water in place of juices, fruited beverages, pop, coffee, etc.
—Fast one day a week.
—Buy grains and beans, the least-expensive food items.

The person committed to nutritional quality as a standard for life and health will find ways to make the food budget work. One such example is our friend, Loretta. Loretta is a single parent with seven children, ages 11 to 18. She lives in low-income housing and has a low-paying job. Yet, because she is committed to the value of good nutrition for her family, she has maintained the Eating Better Lifestyle for many years, even during lean periods such as the last week of the month when there is no money left. If Loretta can do it, we know that it can be done even on the lowest of food budgets.

What About Resources?

> She is like the merchant ships, bringing her food
> from afar. Proverbs 31:14

Availability of fresh fruits and vegetables varies widely by season and by where you live. Certain staples, however, are available almost anywhere there is a market demand. Most supermarkets will carry brown rice, dry beans and peas, fresh fruits and vegetables, buttermilk, yogurt, lowfat milk, chicken, fish, turkey, cheddar and mozzarella cheese, whole wheat flour, rolled oats, unprocessed bran, raisins, dates, honey, peanut butter without sugar or hydrogenated fat, nuts and seeds, olive oil, soy sauce, unsweetened canned pineapple and applesauce, frozen vegetables, and herbs and spices. These items can help you to get a good start. Start reading labels (p. 215) in order to choose the most nutritious food items available. An excellent resource for supermarket purchasing of whole food items and brands in different areas of the country is *The Supermarket Handbook* by Nikki and David Goldbeck. We have also given some mail order resources (pp. 218-20).

Don't hesitate to request your local supermarket manager to carry whole food items such as ground turkey and whole grain breads, for example. Don't be passive about it. Markets are created by customer needs and businesses always want to profit from those needs that rise to the level of demands. Read the labels to find the best available and then request something better, if needed. Sometimes it is easy to overlook what we don't expect to find. For example, Sue's friend Jan, who lives in Washington, D.C., asked us for suggestions where she might purchase whole grains. While visiting her, Sue went shopping one morning at the local supermarket where Jan always shops. There were large bins full of several whole grains and beans. She had just never thought to look for them there! There are wholesome food items in supermarkets and the number will continue to increase as awareness of good nutrition grows.

For other resources check the many categories in the phone book yellow pages that we have listed on page 218. The quality and offerings of health food stores vary widely from vitamin pill shops to exotic herb importers, from the archaic to the leaders in the whole foods industry. Go with the ingredient checklist (p. 199) in hand just to check out what is available. Ask questions. Sue sends her cooking class students with a three-page list. It sometimes creates quite a stir! Many health food store owners specialize in obtaining items unavailable in the supermarkets. Some will special order items in bulk at lower prices. Be aggressive. If we have told you about an ingredient, it's available.

A food co-op can provide good variety at wholesale prices. Co-ops range in sophistication from those which are a simple ministry to a few friends and neighbors to large organizations. In a co-op several people pool their orders to gain the advantage of bulk prices. They work best when a group of people with a common need who know each other on a face-to-face basis follow agreed-upon rules that assure equitable rewards for all.

While we suggest you purchase the most nutritious form of some ingredients, such as low-sodium baking powder and sea salt, recipes may be prepared without them. It is better to start with what you have than not start at all.

12

Helping My Family to Change

> She speaks with wisdom, and faithful instruction
> is on her tongue. She watches over the affairs of her
> household and does not eat the bread of idleness.
> Her children arise and call her blessed; her husband
> also, and he praises her.
>
> Proverbs 31:26-28

Whatever our individual dietary needs may be, most of us must provide food for a family. Short-order cooking for individual tastes and needs is impractical and time-consuming. Therefore, making the change to the Eating Better Lifestyle realistically needs to become a family affair. We have several additional suggestions for helping your family to change in this chapter, but actually many of the things that help to motivate you personally can help to motivate your family as well. Sharing these things in a spirit of love, gentleness, and understanding in a way appropriate to the various ages and temperaments of family members will do a lot to gain acceptance. Pray for the love of Jesus Christ to come through you to your family, because it is as the Holy Spirit changes the heart and renews the mind of each person that true change comes.

If you are married, discuss your desire to make changes with your husband before you start. Pray for wisdom about how to do this, keeping his temperament in mind. If you are not familiar with temperament types, you will find Florence Littauer's books, *Your Personality Tree*, *Personality Plus*, or *How to Get Along With Difficult People*, helpful. While the books do not address food issues specifically, it is very easy to understand that different temperaments will respond differently to food change. If your husband is phlegmatic, for example, he may not get very excited about your adventure, but he will probably be willing to go along with it. If he wants to be more involved in the decision making, cooperate with him and be willing to consider possible limitations to what you can do. If he or any other family member is not like-minded with you, pray for a change of heart and attitudes. What you can explain to children depends on their ages. A good reference for educating children at different ages is Sandy Gooch's, *If You Love Me, Don't Feed Me Junk!* If you are home schooling your children, you have a wonderful opportunity to make the adventure of new foods a part of learning together. Be willing to see what food change means through the eyes of each one. For example, the sanguine child wants to have fun and thrives on compliments. If you have such a child, you might explore what food activities he/she would especially have fun doing. Maybe it is shopping with you, or maybe it is baking cookies. Capitalize on these interests and then freely compliment the child for his/her efforts. The choleric child, the melancholy child, the phlegmatic child, or children with combinations of temperament will react differently from the sanguine.

All family members will want to feel that you care about their reactions to new foods and recipes. Taste enjoyment will be their number-one concern. Sue's family uses a rating scale of 1 to 10 to evaluate each new dish. A rating of 1 means, "Let's please not repeat this one!" A rating of 10 means, "This is really tasty. Let's have it often." A rating anywhere in between gives Sue some indication whether she can improve the recipe by altering some of the ingredients, and how often to serve it. In most cases, if the recipe does not rate an 8 or higher after ingredient adjustments are made, it does not become a part of Sue's recipe file. This one activity of using the rating scale accomplishes several things: 1) It fulfills each person's need to know that his/her opinion matters. 2) It gives Sue an organized plan for building a new recipe file that everyone will enjoy. 3) It takes the pressure off the cook because we all agree that we are not rating the cook's ability, but the recipe. 4) Complaining is minimized because there is assurance that if a recipe is not tasty, it will not become a future part of family meals. If one or two do not like what everyone else agrees is tasty, Sue will make an effort to serve other food with it next time for those who don't care for it. 5) It conveys the idea that this is a family project and that we are experimenting together. When using a rating scale it is a good idea to ask such questions as, "How do you like the taste—is it too bland, too spicy?" "How do you like the texture—the feel of it in your mouth?" "How do you like the smell?" "How does it look to you—is it attractive, colorful?" Keep the perspective that change to better eating is the goal.

Include a special night at least once a month when you serve each person's favorite meal or recipe, improving the nutritional quality of some of the ingredients where you can. If changes don't work well, don't take away the dish until other tasty, but more nutritious dishes, will compensate. You don't have to serve such favorites every day.

Establish some special snack/treat traditions. One mother told us she surprised her children with a small baggie of dates, nuts, and raisins she mixed herself. They thought that was special because she made it special. They didn't know about sugared treats. Another mom shared that her son likes carrot sticks as a treat. Emilie's mother would bake her a potato for an after-school snack. It was a treat and it became a special memory that Emilie passed on to her children. Often we miss the fact that such simple and plain food items give children special pleasure when given in the context of family love.

Mrs. Jones taught Sue to bake cookies (whole grain with honey, of course) just before the children arrived home from school so that the lovely aroma greeted them as they walked in the door. Another welcome treat is a hot carob drink and/or popcorn waiting for the child who has just sloshed home through the pouring rain. You don't need to get into a rut with ordinary snacks. For example, cut out your 100% whole wheat bread with a heart shape, teddy bear, rabbit, or Mickey Mouse cookie cutter. Spread a favorite topping on it such as peanut butter or a light covering of honey-butter. Use raisins as eyes, nose, and mouth. Kids will love it! Take a lesson from television food advertising. Big food companies capture our imagination with clever ideas to promote their products. Let's use our imaginations to advertise our own healthy foods!

Your family will be influenced more by your attitude than by your nutritional pronouncements. It is better not to label your new dishes as "health food," "macrobiotic," or "vegetarian." Avoid a situation where food choices become a battle of the wills. Love changes people, but force seldom does. Here are some Scriptures that will give you real support:

Cheerful attitude—Proverbs 17:22
Don't nag—Proverbs 15:1,17; Proverbs 17:1,14;
 Philippians 2:14; Proverbs 21:23
Apply fruit of the Spirit—Galatians 5:22
Take authority over children—Proverbs 22:6,15;
 Ephesians 6:1
Speak truth in love—Ephesians 4:15
Gentle and quiet spirit—1 Peter 3:4; Philippians 4:5
Not anxious, but prayerful—Philippians 4:6,7
Right motives—1 Thessalonians 1:3; 1 Corinthians 13:13
Hopefulness—Proverbs 22:13; Proverbs 23:18

13

Food Mythology Quiz

Circle T for True, F for False:

T F Vitamin-mineral supplements will make up for the nutrition that is lacking in the food I eat.

T F If I quit eating meat I won't get enough protein.

T F I must use dairy products if I expect to get enough calcium.

T F Carbohydrates are fattening.

T F Fat is fattening.

T F Salt is bad for your health.

T F Honey is no better than sugar.

T F Margarine is healthier than butter.

T F Cholesterol is bad for your health.

T F Raw milk is dangerous.

T F Cooked food is dead food.

T F To lose weight, eat fewer calories.

T F If it's "natural," it's good for you.

All of these statements reflect popular beliefs about food. In the following chapters we will discuss these issues so you can make wiser food choices.

It is the glory of God to conceal a matter; to search out a matter is the glory of kings.

Proverbs 25:2

14

Nutrients on Parade

All things bright and beautiful,
All creatures great and small,
All things wise and wonderful,
The Lord God made them all.
                    —Cecil Frances Alexander, 1818-1895

In addition to oxygen and water the human body needs five groups of known nutrients: carbohydrates, protein, fats, vitamins, and minerals. The first three are called macronutrients and the last two are called micronutrients. We can sort them out easily in the following chart:

Macronutrients: The body uses larger amounts measured in grams. These groups have energy value.
—Carbohydrates: 1 gram = 4 calories
—Protein: 1 gram = 4 calories
—Fats: 1 gram = 9 calories

Micronutrients: The body uses smaller amounts measured in International Units, milligrams, or micrograms (I.U., mg., mcg.). These groups have no energy value.
—Vitamins: about 20 known vitamins
—Minerals: about 17 known minerals

Carbohydrates, fats, proteins, and water are the subtances that food is made of in varying combinations. Vitamins and minerals are contained within the carbohydrates, fats, and proteins. Water contains minerals. All of these nutrients work synergistically in the body for health. The synergism of nutrients means that they work more effectively together than separately. For example, each body cell is like a small factory building the materials necessary for life. This process

59

requires larger amounts of some nutrients and minute amounts of others. Yet every nutrient working together with the others is essential to the health of the whole. Therefore, it is difficult to talk about the functions of each nutrient in an isolated way as if it performed certain things all by itself.

Another way to explain synergism is by Paul's analogy of the human body to the Body of Christ. "Now the body is not made up of one part but of many. . . . The eye cannot say to the hand, 'I don't need you!' And the head cannot say to the feet, 'I don't need you!' . . . If one part suffers, every part suffers with it; if one part is honored, every part rejoices with it" (1 Corinthians 12:14,21,26). Of course, we know that a body can live and function without a hand, an eye, or a foot, but it cannot survive without the head or heart. So it is with food nutrients. Nutrient deficiencies can lead to severe health problems, increased susceptibility to infectious diseases, degenerative diseases, and eventually death. Although we discuss each nutrient group separately for simplicity in the following chapters, we do not want to lose sight of the whole. Each nutrient performs its job fully only in the presence of all the other nutrients supplied in adequate amounts.

Simply stated, God has stored all these nutrients together in a wonderful whole food variety pack!

15

The Challenge of Carbohydrates

"Awk! I can't eat a high carbohydrate diet! I'll get fat!"

Yes, that's right—bread, pastas, cakes, cookies, chips, and candy are fattening! Everybody who's on a diet knows that these foods are out! So carbohydrates must be fattening, right? Wrong! In general, most Americans fail to appreciate carbohydrates because they are confused about what carbohydrates really are.

Carbohydrates are classified in two groups:

1) *simple carbohydrates*:
   sugars present in fruits, honey, maple syrup, sugar cane
   —quick, high-energy foods

2) *complex carbohydrates*:
   starches and dietary fibers present in whole grains, beans and peas, starchy vegetables (potatoes, squash), nuts and seeds
   —slow-releasing high-energy foods
   —dietary fibers and pure water in fresh fruits and vegetables
   —low-energy, cleansing foods

But carbohydrates may also be classified in another way:

1) *unrefined carbohydrates*:
   fresh fruits, fresh vegetables, whole grains, beans and peas, naturally occurring sugars (e.g. honey), nuts and seeds

2) *refined carbohydrates*:
carbohydrate foods stripped of dietary fiber, vitamins, and minerals through processing (e.g. white sugar, white flour, prepackaged foods and mixes made with white sugar and white flour, white rice, degerminated cornmeal, sugary canned fruits and juice)

The entire list—breads, pastas, cakes, cookies, chips, and candy—makes up 50% of our diet in the refined carbohydrate form. We love them, we know they are addictive, and they make us fat! No wonder we are confused about the nutritional value of carbohydrates!

God's design for carbohydrates is much different. He planned them to be our primary source of energy for all the body processes, assistants in metabolizing protein and fat, reservoirs of pure water, wonderful sources of satiating, digestive and fat-regulating fibers, and gold mines of essential vitamins and minerals. These are carbohydrates as man once knew them, and they are the first foods God gave us in the beginning of creation: ". . . I give you every seed-bearing plant on the face of the whole earth and every tree that has fruit with seed in it. They will be yours for food" (Genesis 1:29). Unrefined carbohydrates are the core of the Eating Better Lifestyle. They include both the higher calorie starches and the lower calorie fruits and vegetables. They all contain one nonfattening treasure—dietary fiber.

16

Making Friends with Fiber

Great are the works of the LORD; they are pon-
dered by all who delight in them.

Psalm 111:2

Incredible as it may seem, the lack of just one food nutrient—dietary fiber—contributes to tragic suffering in America.
Millions are burdened by digestive disorders, cancers, heart
disease, diabetes, and obesity. Fiber is a God-given resource.
Remove it from our foods and we suffer.

Kinds of Fiber

Actually fiber is not yet classified as a nutrient. Part of the
fiber in plant foods was discovered in 1887 and labeled as
crude fiber. Many food package labels list crude fiber. In 1972
dietary fiber was discovered. It includes several different
types of fiber. There is three to seven times more dietary fiber
than crude fiber in foods.

Dietary fiber includes water-soluble fibers and insoluble
fibers. The water-soluble fibers are gums and pectins. The
best food sources of gums are oats, especially the bran, and
all beans and peas (legumes). The best sources of pectin are
apples, citrus fruits, carrots, cauliflower, squash, green beans,
cabbage, dried peas, strawberries, and potatoes. The insoluble fibers are cellulose, hemicelluloses, and lignin. The best
sources of these fibers are whole grains including whole
wheat, especially wheat bran. Apples, carrots, green and
wax beans, peppers, cabbage, broccoli, brussels sprouts, and
young peas are also excellent sources of cellulose. Mature
vegetables, strawberries, eggplant, pears, green beans, and
radishes are high in lignin. Most vegetables, grains, beans

and peas, and nuts and seeds contain more than one dietary fiber in varying proportions. The amounts and effects of these fibers can vary with the stage of growth, the age of the plants, and the way they are prepared.

Functions of Fiber

Dietary fibers perform different functions in the human body. Insoluble fibers add bulk by absorbing water in the digestive track. This speeds up the transit time of food through the digestive system. Lack of bulk contributes to constipation, hiatus hernia, gallstones, diverticulosis, spastic colon, hemorrhoids, varicose veins, diarrhea, colitis, appendicitis, and colon cancer. Insoluble fibers may also help to remove toxins, pesticide residues, and carcinogenic bacteria from the body.

Soluble fibers, and also lignin, help to regulate blood cholesterol and triglyceride levels, decrease fat absorption, and moderate wide swings in blood sugar levels. These processes are important for the prevention and moderation of hypoglycemia, diabetes, heart disease, and weight. The satiety value of fiber, the feeling of being full, also assists weight control. Fewer calories of high-fiber foods are more filling and also require more chewing. The "I've had enough signals" will reach the brain before you have overeaten. In addition "carbohydrate goes through different pathways from fat—pathways that burn off more calories"[1] Of course, we are talking about unrefined carbohydrate calories and not white sugar and white flour!

Considerable research lends support to these benefits. The British medical journal, *Lancet*, September 4, 1982, reports the findings of a ten-year Netherlands study performed on 871 men. The death rate among the men on low-fiber diets was four times higher from heart disease, three times higher from cancer, and three times higher from all causes than that of the men who ate about 37 grams of dietary fiber per day. Disease declined proportionately with the increase of dietary fiber. Studies of countries reveal that societies with high-fiber diets consistently have significantly lower rates of heart disease, cancer (especially colon cancer), and diabetes. What wonders to perform! But how much dietary fiber do we need?

Ways to Increase Fiber

The American Diet includes only 5 to 20 grams of dietary fiber per day. Recommendations range from 25 to 40 grams. Aim toward 40 grams. Emphasizing one kind of fiber, such as the insoluble fibers, by sprinkling wheat bran into everything or taking high-fiber food supplements is inadequate. The best way to get the full range of dietary fibers is to make 45% to 65% of your calorie intake* unrefined carbohydrates. Include a variety of fresh vegetables, fruits, whole grains, beans and peas, and nuts and seeds. The chart following gives the approximate dietary fiber in these foods. To ensure that our bodies get the benefits of dietary fiber variety, we also need to drink plenty of water, spread fiber foods throughout all the meals of the day, and eat lots of raw foods. Cooking vegetables does not decrease the fiber, but stir-frying and steaming seem to be the best preparation methods. To avoid the problems of gas or diarrhea ease into a high-fiber diet. It takes time for the digestive system to become accustomed to an increase in fiber.

You may read that high fiber can prevent some important minerals from being absorbed by the body. Don't worry about this. It can happen initially as you adjust, but in the long run, a wide variety of plant foods and a level of 30 to 40 grams of dietary fiber should not create this problem.

If you have any chronic health condition such as colon problems or diabetes, it is important to consult your physician about the best way to gradually add dietary fiber to your diet.

Happy fibrous eating!

---

*See Calorie Chart, p. 69.
Example: 45% to 65% of 1,800 Calories = 810 to 1,170 Calories
 (.45 x 1,800 = 810, .65 x 1,800 = 1,170)

Dietary Fiber in Foods

Amounts listed supply about 4 grams of dietary fiber each.*

Whole Grains, Flours, Breads, Cereals	Amount
barley, uncooked	1¼ cup
bran, oat, dry	3 Tbsp.
bran, wheat, dry	¼ cup
bulgur wheat (Ala)	½ cup dry
cornmeal, stoneground	¼ cup
corn tortillas	10
Grape Nuts	¼ cup
millet cereal, cooked	1 cup
Nutri-Grain, Kellogg's (Almond Raisin)	1 cup
popped corn	2½ cups
rice, brown	1½ cup
rice, white	5 cups
rolled oats, uncooked	½ cup
Roman Meal, uncooked	⅓ cup
rye bread	2½ slices
rye crackers, wafers	5
rye flour, dark	¼ cup
shredded wheat	2 large biscuits
shredded wheat, spoon size	1 cup
Wheatena, cooked	1¼ cup
Wheaties	2 cups
whole wheat bread	2½ slices
whole wheat flour	2 cups
Total (General Mills)	2 cups

Legumes (Dry Beans, Peas, cooked)	
black beans	¼ cup
black-eyed peas	¼ cup
broad beans	1 cup
garbanzos (chickpeas)	⅓ cup
kidney beans	1⅛ cup
lentils	⅓ cup
lima beans	1½ cup
pinto beans	⅔ cup
split peas	⅓ cup
soybeans	1½ cup
white beans	½ cup

Fruits, uncooked	
apple with skin	1 (4 oz.)
applesauce (cooked)	1¼ cup

*No standard laboratory measurement of dietary fiber has been established. Different tables give slightly varying measures in different foods. Dietary fiber data is also given for all recipes in the *Eating Better Cookbooks* (see p. 287 for information).

Fruits, uncooked cont.

avocado, 10 oz.	1
bananas, medium	2
blackberries	½ cup
blueberries	4 cups
cherries, sweet	44
cranberries	3 cups
dates	1 cup
figs, dried, small	5
grapefruit	2 halves
orange, small-medium	2
pears, small with skin	2
plums, small	5
pineapple	2½ cups
prunes, dried	3
raisins	6 Tbsp.
raspberries	⅔ cup
strawberries	1 cup
tangerines, medium	2

Vegetables, uncooked

bean sprouts	1¼ cup
cabbage	2 cups
carrot, large	1
cauliflower	2 cups
celery stalks (4 oz.)	3
cucumber, 10-inch (8 oz.)	2½ cups
lettuce	4-5 cups
radishes	1⅓ cup
spinach	4-5 leaves

Vegetables, cooked

artichoke, medium	1
asparagus	1 cup
beans, green snap	1 cup
beets	1 cup
broccoli	1 cup
brussels sprouts	½ cup
cabbage	1½ cup
carrots	1 cup
collards	1 cup
corn	½ cup
cauliflower	2 cups
eggplant	2 cups
kale	1 cup
onions	1¼ cup
parsnips	½ cup
peas, green	½ cup
potatoes	1 cup
baked, small-medium	1
rutabagas	1¼ cup
spinach	1 cup
squash, summer	1 cup
squash, winter	1⅛ cup

Vegetables, cooked cont.

sweet potato, large (yam, U.S. variety)	1
tomatoes	1 cup
turnips	1 cup
zucchini	1 cup

Nuts and Seeds

almonds, slivered	1½ cups
whole	40
cashews	1⅛ cup
coconut	¾ cup
peanuts with skins	1¼ cup
pecans	16
sesame seeds, whole	½ cup
sunflower seeds	¾ cup
walnuts	2¼ Tbsp.

Calorie Chart*

Use this chart to learn what foods are low-, moderate-, and high-calorie. "Accounting for every calorie" is not essential to the Eating Better Lifestyle. The amounts listed are approximate ranges only.

Count 0 Calories for Average Serving Size

- celery
- cucumber
- lettuce
- mushrooms
- onions
- radishes
- raw spinach
- alfalfa sprouts
- bean sprouts, raw
- mustard
- soy sauce
- vinegar
- lemon juice
- lime juice
- herb or black tea
- decaffeinated coffee

Count 50 Calories

Fruits
½ cup:
- grapes
- blackberries
- blueberries
- loganberries
- pineapple
- cherries
- unsweetened applesauce
- unsweetened canned fruits

1 cup:
- strawberries
- raspberries
- melons

Count 50 Calories

Pieces:
- ½ grapefruit
- 1 peach
- 1 fig
- 1 orange
- 1 tangelo
- 1 tangerine
- 1 quince
- 1 kiwi fruit
- 2-3 dates
- 2-3 plums
- 3-4 apricots

Vegetables:
½ cup:
- corn
- peas
- canned tomatoes
- winter squash
- ripe olives
- pasta or tomato sauce

1 cup:
- cabbage (raw)
- dark leafy greens (cooked)
  spinach, collards, kale,
  turnip, mustard
- bean sprouts (cooked)
- okra
- beets
- broccoli
- brussels sprouts
- cauliflower (cooked)
- carrots
- rutabaga
- eggplant

---

*For more specific calorie counts use the *Eating Better Cookbooks* (see p. 287 for information).

Count 50 Calories

Vegetables cont.
2 cups:
cauliflower (raw)
beet greens (cooked)
cabbage (cooked)
zucchini
vegetable salads, most

Pieces:
1 artichoke
1 large carrot
1 large tomato
8-12 asparagus spears

Breads, Crackers, Cereals:
1 cup puffed cereals
1 cup plain popcorn
6-inch corn tortilla
2 brown rice cakes
2 triple Rykrisp

Nuts and Seeds:
1 Tbsp. chopped (most)
2-3 Tbsp. coconut

Dairy Products:
2 Tbsp. Parmesan cheese
1 Tbsp. cream cheese
1½ Tbsp. sour cream
½ cup nonfat plain yogurt
1 medium egg

Sweets and Spreads:
1 Tbsp. honey or fructose
1 Tbsp. jam
1 Tbsp. maple syrup
1 Tbsp. sorghum
3 Tbsp. ketchup

Count 100 Calories

Fruits:
1 nectarine
1 small mango
1 small papaya
1 pear
1 small persimmon
1 pomegranate
1 small banana
¼ avocado
fruit salads, most

Count 100 Calories

Fruits, Dried:
¼ cup raisins
¼ cup dried apricots
5 prunes, dried
1 slice dried pineapple

Fruit Juices:
¾ to 1 cup

Vegetables:
5 oz. (small) Irish potato
⅓ cup sweet potato
⅓ cup yam (U.S. variety)
7-inch ear corn

Breads, Cereals:
½ cup brown rice (cooked)
½ cup bulgur (cooked)
½ cup pasta (cooked)
macaroni, noodles, spaghetti
1 oz. serving cold or hot cereals (¼ to 1 cup—check cereal box)
1 slice (1.5 oz.) whole grain bread
1 whole wheat tortilla
1 whole wheat pita bread
½ whole wheat English muffin
1 whole grain dinner roll
4 (1 oz.) Akmak whole wheat crackers
1 cookie
gelatin dessert

Dairy Products:
¼ cup (1 oz.) cheddar cheese
⅓ cup ricotta cheese
½ cup:
lowfat cottage cheese
whole milk
lowfat plain yogurt
lowfat vanilla yogurt
nonfat fruit yogurt
tofu
¾ cup (6 oz.):
buttermilk
lowfat milk
1 large or extra-large egg

Meats:
⅓ cup tuna

Count 100 Calories

Meats cont.
4 oz. serving lean fish:
    bass
    haddock
    halibut
    ocean perch
    pollock
    snapper
    cod
    flounder
3 oz. fish:
    bluefish
    carp
    catfish
    swordfish

Fats:
1 tablespoon:
    butter
    vegetable oil
    mayonnaise
    peanut butter

Count 150 Calories

1 whole grain muffin

Count 200 Calories

Meat, Fish, Poultry:
4 oz. serving fatty fish:
    herring
    mackerel
    salmon
    shad
    whitefish
3.5 oz. or ¾ cup:
    chicken
    turkey
    ½ cup ground turkey
4 oz. serving red meats:
    beef chuck
    flank steak
    round steak
    lean ground beef
    leg of lamb
    meat loaf

Nuts and Seeds:
    ¼ cup chopped

Count 200 Calories

Sweets:
    ¼ cup maple syrup

Dry Wine:
    1 cup

Count 200 to 400 Calories

(check amounts of individual recipes)
    casseroles, most
    sandwiches, most
    soups, most
    cakes and desserts, most

Count 300 Calories

Meats, red—4 oz. serving:
    rump roast
    sirloin steak
    regular ground beef
    lamb, shoulder, chops

Breads:
    4 whole grain pancakes
    average serving waffles

Sweet Wine:
    1 cup

Count 400 Calories

meats, red—4 oz. serving:
    rib roast
    club steak
    porterhouse steak
    T-bone steak
    1 piece pie (⅛ pie)

Count Over 400 Calories (highest)

average serving:
    quiches
    bean burritos
    tostada, meatless or not
    pizza
    beef or turkey burgers
    some cheesy and/or meaty casseroles
    1 piece double-crust pie (⅛ pie)

17

Plenty of Protein!

How many are your works, O LORD! In wisdom
you made them all.

Psalm 104:24

Depending on weight, our bodies need 40 to 60 grams of
protein daily. Protein, the primary building material for the
body, helps in forming the hormones and enzymes, in main-
taining water balance and acid/base balance in the body, in
forming mother's milk, and in clotting of blood. Surely it is
one of our Lord's nutrient marvels!

Fortunately, protein deficiency is uncommon in the United
States. In fact, the American Diet contains twice as much
protein as needed. The concern that meat or dairy products
are essential for adequate protein intake is unfounded. Getting plenty of protein into meals through a variety of whole
foods in good balance is very easy—much easier than getting
enough dietary fiber in and getting excessive fat out! How do
we do it?

The protein that our bodies need consists of a combination
of 22 amino acids. They are called "the building blocks" of the
protein molecule. Eight of these are called essential amino
acids because they cannot be manufactured in the body. They
are tryptophan, leucine, isoleucine, lysine, valine, threo-
nine, methionine, and cystine. A ninth, histidine, is essential for young children and possibly for adults. Practically
every food has some of the essential amino acids, even fruits,
although they have the least. Vegetables contain a little more
and grains, beans, nuts, and seeds are even higher. All of
these unrefined carbohydrates are called incomplete proteins

because none of them adequately supplies all eight essential amino acids. In contrast, meat, fish, poultry, eggs, and dairy products do contain all eight and are therefore called complete proteins.

It has been thought that all eight essential amino acids must be eaten at the same meal to get the full benefit of them all. That's why we have come to understand that we need animal foods for protein. Yet all of the essential amino acids are supplied in our carbohydrate foods when we eat them in a good variety. Some combinations of incomplete protein will make complete protein dishes. For example, grains are low in lysine but beans are not. When the two are combined, complete protein is formed. In addition, when complete protein foods such as milk, eggs, or cheese are combined with incomplete protein foods such as grains, the protein value of the grains is increased. Combinations of complex carbohydrates that make complete protein are:

> *grains and beans*—such as chili and cornbread, peanut butter and bread, lentils and rice, baked beans and brown bread
> *grains and dark leafy greens*—such as rice pilaf and spinach salad
> *grains and dairy products*—such as macaroni and cheese, toasted cheese sandwich, muffins or pancakes made with milk and eggs
> *beans and sesame or sunflower seeds*—such as garbanzo spread or falafel, kidney beans and sunflower seeds in a salad

These are called complimentary protein combinations. The need for these combinations in one meal has probably been overrated. Actually, including these foods regularly at any time in our meals in any combination is sufficient to supply adequate protein. The key is variety. In countries where variety is unavailable, protein deficiencies can occur. Communities that rely on corn, for example, can be deficient in lysine. A high-lysine corn has been developed in recent to work toward meeting such needs as this. We would do well to think seriously about those who are in much greater need than ourselves. Then we will begin to be thankful for the incredible variety that is ours!

18

The Slippery Subject of Fats!

In days gone by men argued, "Is the earth really round or flat?" Today it concerns the safety of: "What kind and how much fat?"

Have you ever tried to explain something simply and clearly and then realized that your explanations raised more questions than answers? So it is with the subject of fats! If ever new products have been promoted on fear, this is it. Cholesterol is practically synonymous with sin. Advertising provides simple, and often wrong, solutions.

Nutritional research, however, is quite a different matter. There are more questions than answers. The result is that you and I see contradiction and controversy that leaves us confused. What are we going to do? First, let's find out what fat is good for, what kinds of fats there are, and then which ones are our best choices.

We've put some foods that involve the fat issue into other chapters—meats, eggs, and dairy products. Therefore, we won't discuss these foods in much detail in this chapter, but will focus on the almost exclusively concentrated fats—vegetable oils and butter.

We Need Some Fat!

First of all, fat in itself is not bad. Our bodies need fat to transport the fat-soluble vitamins (A, D, E, and K), to convert carotene from plant foods to vitamin A, to protect vital organs, to regulate temperature, to provide a concentrated source of energy, to provide the essential fatty acid (linoleic acid), to satiate hunger, and to add wonderful flavor to many dishes.

Even cholesterol fat is not bad. Cholesterol is a necessary part of all body cells, especially nerve, brain, blood, and liver cells. It assists in nutrient and waste transport in and out of the cells, assists in the forming of bile and vital hormones, and lubricates the skin. Our bodies use much more cholesterol fat than our food provides, and manufacture what needed cholesterol fat is not consumed in food. We do not want to cast fat aside, but to regulate it.

What Kinds of Fat Are There?

Just as with dietary fiber, all fats are not in the same form. The four basic known forms of fat are polyunsaturated, saturated, monosaturated, and cholesterol. No oils from plant foods contain cholesterol. Some vegetable oils are high in polyunsaturates with less saturated and monosaturated fats, such as safflower, sunflower, corn, and soybean oils. Some are more highly saturated such as cottonseed (26%), palm oil (51%), palm kernel oil (86%), and coconut oil (92%). These latter, more highly saturated oils, are primarily used in prepackaged processed foods of all kinds and also for frying in many restaurants and fast-food outlets because they are less expensive. Olive oil, peanut oil, and the fat in avocados are called monosaturated oils because they contain a higher percentage of monosaturated fat. All animal foods contain saturated fat, unsaturated fat, and cholesterol. Among animal foods, fish are lowest in saturated fat and cholesterol, and contain valuable polyunsaturated fatty acids.

How Fat Can Affect Weight Control

The confusion and controversy surrounding these forms of fat involves their various effects on health in special regard to cancers, heart disease, and weight control. The least confusing issue is the effect of fats on weight control. All fats, no matter what form, contain nine calories per gram, twice as many calories as a gram of protein or carbohydrate. A high-fat diet, very simply, adds too many calories too easily for most people, especially in combination with a refined carbohydrate diet that contains inadequate dietary fibers. Limiting overall intake of fat of all kinds is a very effective way to control calorie levels.

Other Problems with Animal Fats and Oils

Many research studies have shown a correlation between heart disease and fats. The most well-established link to date is that diets that are higher in saturated fats do raise blood cholesterol levels, a leading contributor to heart-disease risk. This is the reason that we have been cautioned to reduce meats and dairy products and encouraged to use more vegetable oils, because they are much higher in polyunsaturated fat. Other research shows that polyunsaturates reduce blood cholesterol. Yet, other studies indicate that too much polyunsaturated oil may lead to certain forms of cancer. The reason for this is that highly polyunsaturated vegetable oils go rancid easily. Rancid oils in the body, simply stated, are carcinogenic. Refinement of oils extracts the vitamin E, which acts as a natural preservative, and the heating of oils in cooking can compound the risk of rancidity. Vegetable oils really are a refined food. They are the highly concentrated fat portion of nuts and seeds divorced from their original whole food complex carbohydrate form with all the original dietary fiber, vitamins, minerals, and other unknown nutrients. The more refined an oil, the fewer original nutrients remain. Not even cold-pressed oils contain a healthy level of the original vitamin E that acts as a preservative in high-fat plant foods. We recommend using either cold-pressed oils or unrefined oils (very strong-tasting) in limited amounts. These may be purchased at health food stores. All oils should be kept under refrigeration.

What About Hydrogenated Vegetable Fat, Margarine, and Butter?

Added to the extraction of nutrients in oil processing is the frequent hydrogenation of fat. Hydrogenation adds an extra hydrogen molecule to give oils a longer shelf life. Oils lightly hydrogenated will be thicker, yet still liquid at room temperature. Heavily hydrogenated oils will be solid at room temperature. Vegetable shortenings and margarines are hydrogenated. Hydrogenation increases the saturation of fats. Vegetable shortenings are often made from more highly saturated fats to begin with, such as Crisco which is made from hydrogenated soybean and palm oil (51% saturated). Hydrogenation also changes the natural *cis* form of fatty acids into *trans* fatty acids. Some nutritionists maintain that the body cannot utilize the *trans* form of fatty acids. According to Warren N. Levin, M.D., member of the International Academy of Preventive Medicine, "These trans-fatty acids do not fit into the body machinery and tend to 'gum up the works.' "[1] Therefore, Dr. Levin recommends butter over margarine, although butter is a saturated fat. Carlton Fredericks, Ph.D., also wrote in regard to margarine in "Hotline to Health," *Prevention* (December, 1980, p. 39), "A recent report in the *Journal of Nutrition* (October, 1979, pp. 1759-65) warns that excessive intake of trans fats tends to aggravate existing deficiencies in essential fatty acids." We are inclined to agree with these findings on the basis that man's chemical alterations of real foods repeatedly have been found wanting in their effects upon human health. There may be quite a bit we don't know concerning the effects of trans fatty acids on human health that we will wish later that we did know. For these reasons we recommend not using vegetable shortening or margarine.

In the meantime, as we have been faced with this fat dilemma, modern research is turning up exciting new information about olive oil and fish. Conservative scientific researchers are cautious, however, and tell us that final proof is not yet available.

Olive Oil

New studies indicate that olive oil, a monosaturated fat, is also effective in lowering blood cholesterol levels without having the dangers in relationship to cancers that polyunsaturated fats do. In addition, olive oil assists bowel regularity, and ". . . .is easily digested, imparting a soothing and healing influence to the digestive tract. This healing and cleansing effect is due to the high content of potassium and also sodium and calcium."[2] Olive oil is the primary vegetable oil used regularly in Mediterranean countries. People in this area do not suffer the high incidence of heart disease that we do in America. We are quite excited about these findings. Olive oil has been spoken of well in the Bible: "Observe the commands of the LORD your God, walking in his ways and revering him. For the LORD your God is bringing you into a good land—a land with streams and pools of water, with springs flowing in the valleys and hills; a land with wheat and barley, vines and fig trees, pomegranates, olive oil and honey . . . " (Deuteronomy 8:6-9), and ". . . every one of you will eat from his own vine and fig tree and drink water from his own cistern, until I come and take you to a land like your own, a land of grain and new wine, a land of bread and vineyards, a land of olive trees and honey. Choose life and not death!" (2 Kings 18:31b,32).

We do not yet know for certain if the virgin form of olive oil is better for the body than the less expensive pure olive oil. But chances are good that virgin olive oil is better. True virgin olive oil is difficult to find, however, and pure olive oil is expensive enough. The expense of olive oil is really a blessing in disguise as this should prevent most of us from using too much of it! We believe that reducing the polyunsaturated vegetable oil used in our diet and replacing some of it with olive oil is a wise idea. Try Emilie's gourmet Olive Oil Vinegar Dressing (p. 276) that she learned from her famous Viennese chef father.

Fat Fish Story

The new discovery in fish is EPA and DHA (called omega-3 fatty acids), two polyunsaturated fatty acids that lower blood cholesterol and triglycerides. Fatty fish are highest in EPA and DHA, and include mackerel, salmon, blue fish, sardines, mullet, rainbow trout, lake trout, herring, tuna, sable fish, shad, butterfish, and pompano. No one knows yet how much fish will accomplish these health effects, but one suggestion is two to four fish meals a week in contrast to the average American's one fish meal a week. Fish is easily digested and very high in protein. Weston A. Price, D.D.S., who toured the world to extensively study the health condition of over 100 tribal groups in the 1940's, reported in his book *Nutrition and Physical Degeneration* that the strongest, most energetic people groups were those who had access to seafoods. The Eskimos who have lived on a very high fat whale meat diet have not suffered from heart disease. The Japanese whose diets are high in seafoods have also enjoyed a low incidence of heart trouble.

Eating even one more fish meal a week than we now eat will count for better health. See page 83 for some cautions on the kinds of fish to choose.

Cholesterol-Lowering Foods

Some interesting studies reveal that certain foods can lower blood cholesterol levels. For example, a group of men was given 18 tablespoons of oat bran a day for ten days. Their blood cholesterol drop averaged 18%.[3] Most people would not consume on a regular daily diet so much of any one food. We do not yet know how much of any one food or a combination of foods in a normal diet might assist in regulating cholesterol levels. Foods that may contribute to normal blood cholesterol levels, however, include garlic, onions, avocados, eggplant, seeds, cabbage, soybeans, peanuts, oats, oat bran, beans, yams, and barley. Both dietary fibers and other properties in these foods are of value. There may be other whole foods, as well, that we may discover that contribute to the body's ability to handle fats properly. All these foods may work together synergistically (p. 59) for our health.

A Fat Menu to Keep You From Slipping

Include more fish, especially the fatty kind.
Use a little olive oil,
and leave some of those polys* behind!
Let the hydroges* on the shelf remain—
that means the shortening,
the "partiallys,"*
and the mar-gar-ine.
Use nuts and seeds often,
but fresh and few;
chew them well for great taste,
crunch, and nutrients, too!
Opt for real butter, but just a tad;
Keep fats below 30% of cals*
And you'll be glad!

And maybe, one day,
Just as the earth went
from flat to round,
All the fat facts you need
will finally abound!

---

*polyunsaturated fats, hydrogenated fats, partially hydrogenated fats, calories. Keep concentrated vegetable and butter fats to 1 to 2 tablespoons per day.

19

Is Meat a Menace
to Your Health?

> Do not join those who drink too much wine or
> gorge themselves on meat, for drunkards and glut-
> tons become poor, and drowsiness clothes them in
> rags.
>
> Proverbs 23:20,21

Problems

Americans consume 30% of the world's animal protein, yet
we are only 7% of the world's population. Worldwide, the
more affluent a society becomes and the more influenced by
Western civilization, the more meat-centered it becomes. The
meat-centered diet reflects the belief that we must have it to
meet our protein needs. In fact, many homemakers don't
know how to plan a menu without it. In the meantime vegetarians are enjoying less incidence of diabetes, high blood
pressure, osteoporosis, high estrogen levels and gallstones in
women, high blood cholesterol levels, heart disease, and
hormone-related cancer in men (such as prostate).

The quality of our meat is not what it once was a short 40
years ago. Beef used to be a lean 5% to 10% fat when cattle
were range-fed on grasses and matured over two to three
years. Today high-energy feeds and 18 months of fast growth
marbleizes the beef with over 30% saturated fat. Meat production has become a huge economic enterprise requiring over
2,700 drugs including antibiotics, hormones, tranquilizers,
and pesticides. More drugs are used by cattlemen than by
medical doctors. Chemical residues inevitably remain in the
meat and cannot be cooked out. An excellent reference that
thoroughly discusses the problems with all animal foods,
including eggs and dairy products, in both production and
nutritional value, is *The New Vegetarian* by Gary Null.

Among the food groups, animal products are the most highly susceptible to bacterial contamination. In fact salmonella contamination is so high that testing for it has not been considered worth the time. The USDA reported recently that "Nearly four out of every ten chickens sold to consumers are contaminated by salmonella . . ."[1] Millions suffer yearly from these contaminated meats. For example, between 1971 and 1983 there were over 15 million estimated associations of salmonella illness with meat and poultry.[2] Scientists estimate that about 30% of the 69 million to 275 million cases of diarrhea that occur each year result from food contamination.[3] Although salmonella can be destroyed through proper cooking, bacteria can be carried from hands contaminated with infected raw meat to other foods. The most frequent victims are the elderly, the sick, the unborn, and infants.

Pork and shellfish have always been scavengers by nature. That means that they act like living garbage cans. High quality feed notwithstanding, pigs cannot be divorced from their scavenger nature. They will eat their own feces even in the most carefully controlled situations.

The danger of pork, improperly cooked, has been understood as trichinosis, caused by a parasite that can enter the body through pork that has been eaten. *The Albany Democrat-Herald* (Saturday, October 11, 1980) carried an article entitled, "Trichinosis now affects only about 2% of U.S. population, Center for Disease Control reports." Two percent of the American population is approximately 4½ million people. "Most don't even know they are infected and the cases never are reported."

Industrial wastes poured into lakes, rivers, and oceans are slowly contaminating our fish supply as well. Freshwater fish from inland lakes and rivers are the most contaminated, especially with PCB's. Swordfish and carp contain the highest mercury levels. Deep ocean fish and smaller fish are less likely to be contaminated. Pregnant women especially, should avoid high levels of both PCB's and mercury. Fresh fish can also be sprayed with chemicals to help preserve freshness before it is sold.

Historically people have eaten very small amounts of meat compared to complex carbohydrates. Even at the turn of the century Americans ate less than half the meat eaten today although their protein intake was about the same. Animal foods are more difficult to digest than plant foods. Fish is the easiest meat to digest, followed by poultry.

Solutions

Our recipes and menus in Part 6 give you ideas for both meatless meals and meals with small amounts of meat. We suggest a goal of serving three meat meals a week at most. Replace red meats with fish and poultry. You might serve chicken one evening, turkey or lamb another evening, fish a third evening. Fish might be served more frequently, however. Replace regular ground beef with ground turkey. It is lower in calories and fat, and poultry is easier for the body to digest. Ground turkey contains turkey skin, however, so it is higher in fat than turkey dark meat and light meat. Aim for serving smaller amounts of meat in stir-fry dishes and casseroles.

Try to purchase meats that have been grown without drugs. These may be labeled "organically grown." Call your local health food store, a local food co-op, and check resources (p. 218). Do not purchase beef or chicken livers unless grown without drugs. The liver is a dumping ground for toxic residues. Use only fresh or frozen meats and not processed meats with preservatives such as nitrites or nitrates and refined sugars added.

When you prepare meats, wash your hands thoroughly before handling other food, dishes, utensils, or cleaning supplies. Cut meats on a hard plastic cutting board that you can wash in the dishwasher. Use a different board for cutting other foods. Thaw all your meats in the refrigerator or the microwave. Don't leave any meats, cooked or raw, standing at room temperature over two hours. Bacteria multiply rapidly between 40° F. and 140° F. Cook poultry and meats thoroughly without interrupting the process.

To reduce fat content, remove skin from chicken and turkey. Trim all the visible fat from meats. Bake, broil, or fry in non-stick pans and drain off all excess fat. Charcoal broiling produces high amounts of benzoprene residue, a carcinogen related to leukemia and stomach cancer.[4]

It is a fact that on any given day, 80% of Americans see very little, if any, fresh produce on their plates. The American Diet Chart (p. 28) illustrates this. Gary Null in *The New Vegetarian* reminds us that "Meat eaters' diets are likely to be much more restricted than vegetarians' diets. . . . When meat is the center of the meal, contributions from other food groups (grains, legumes, fruits, and vegetables) are often kept to minimum servings."[5] By reducing our dependency on meats as the focus of our menu planning, we are free to enjoy a greater variety of God's cornucopia of wholefoods.

20

Eggs—Ample of Controversy!

> As an inexpensive source of good nutrition,
> there is nothing more glorious than the egg.
>
> Edward Ahrens

The controversy and confusion over eggs focuses on the high cholesterol content of egg yolks. Media advertising, news articles, magazines, nutrition books, cookbooks, doctors, and nutritionists would have us believe that food cholesterol raises blood cholesterol. Yet there is no adequate research to substantiate this claim. Researchers are not agreed at all on this issue. The classic study that relates egg yolk cholesterol to blood cholesterol was conducted in 1913 by Nikolai Anichkov, a Russian pathologist, on rabbits. He fed rabbits the equivalent to human consumption of 60 eggs per day. The rabbits developed cholesterol deposits on their arteries. But rabbits are total vegetarians and do not eat eggs. "There is nothing in their metabolism to handle eggs."[1]

No human study shows a clear relationship between food cholesterol content and blood cholesterol, whereas research does indicate a clearer relationship to total fat consumption, especially to saturated fat. Yet eggs are lower in saturated fat than both meat and poultry, about the same as lowfat yogurt, and contain 1/3 of the amount that is in 1/4 cup (1 oz.) of cheddar cheese.

Advertising and popular news articles repeatedly reinforce the notion that food cholesterol raises blood cholesterol levels. "No cholesterol" labels are printed on vegetable oils and advertised everywhere. The message is effectively communicated: "Cholesterol in foods must be bad!"

Time Magazine, March 26, 1984, reported the most extensive research project ever conducted on cholesterol in medical history. This project has been declared ". . . a turning point in cholesterol-heart-disease research,"[2] because it clearly demonstrated that high blood cholesterol contributes to heart disease and cardiac deaths. Ten years and $150 million were spent on 3,806 men, ages 35 to 39 with cholesterol levels of 265 mg. A cholesterol-lowering drug was used in the study. Those receiving the drug experienced an 8.5% drop in cholesterol, 19% fewer heart attacks, and 24% fewer cardiac deaths. Yet nothing was changed in their diets. The study had nothing to do with cholesterol content of any foods.

The editors of *Time Magazine* placed a "sad-face" picture on the front cover of its March 26, 1984 issue using two fried eggs for eyes and a slice of bacon for the mouth, with an overcaption of "Cholesterol . . . And Now the Bad News." On page 56 the article was entitled, "Hold the Eggs and Butter." The message conveyed to the reader was that "Eggs and butter contribute to heart disease." Yet the research project reviewed by *Time* had nothing to do with the effects of food on cholesterol! This kind of media influence confuses important nutritional issues for the American public. Of this research project Edward Ahrens, researcher at Rockefeller University, said, "Since this was basically a drug study we can conclude nothing about diet; such extrapolation is unwarranted, unscientific and wishful thinking."[3]

Only 20% to 30% of our cholesterol comes from food. Our bodies manufacture the rest. There are many other influences on blood cholesterol levels besides total fat intake, such as exercise, stress, inherited genes, prepackaged foods high in fats and refined carbohydrates, lack of dietary fiber, and inadequate vitamins and minerals. Rather than focus on egg yolks as a dietary disaster, we should develop a balance of real whole foods.

Eggs are a real food. They can readily be used in baking and a couple of times a week for meals. Two breakfasts or an egg main dish will not raise the total fat intake to over 30% of calories. Eggs are our best protein source because their amino acid pattern most nearly matches that needed for human growth and health.[4] They are excellent sources of trace minerals, unsaturated fatty acids, iron, phosphorus, vitamin B-complex, A, E, K, and even some D. Most of these reside in the egg yolk! Yolks also are the highest food source of choline, a component of lecithin that assists in keeping cholesterol liquid in the bloodstream. There is some question as to whether the lecithin is effective in this way, however.

If you do not want to eat egg yolks or are allergic to eggs, be encouraged. There are easy alternatives! You can use two egg whites in place of a whole egg in almost any baking recipe. Unfortunately that wastes the egg yolks, so we prefer using ¼ cup tofu in place of an egg. Mixing it in the blender with other liquid ingredients works best. We also have a wonderful recipe for Tofu Scramble (p. 253) and Tofu Salad Spread (p. 267) as alternatives to scrambled eggs and egg salad. We discourage the use of egg substitutes. If you cannot find a real food to give taste pleasure, we recommend doing without.

Consider the value of fertile eggs. Fertile eggs come from hens, living with roosters, that are allowed to grow and peck on the ground. They receive no drugs as chickens raised in close quarters do. We don't really know what the nutritional difference between fertile eggs and sterile eggs is even though some people make claims for the nutritional superiority of fertile eggs. The clearest advantage is that fertile eggs are free of chemical residues. In general, fertile eggs also taste fresher but are also slightly more expensive. Many health food stores carry them. People who raise their own chickens also often sell them.

Mankind has eaten eggs for centuries. Even Job ate eggs: ". . . is there flavor in the white of an egg? I refuse to touch it; such food makes me ill" (Job 6:6,7). Yet heart disease was not reported in scientific literature until 1896.[5] You decide. We still believe eggs are an economical blessing from God given to us to enjoy in moderation.

21

Are Dairy Products Deadly?

> The virgin . . . will call him Immanuel. He will
> eat curds and honey when he knows enough to
> reject the wrong and choose the right. . . . In that
> day, a man will keep alive a young cow and two
> goats. And because of the abundance of the milk
> they give, he will have curds to eat. All who remain
> in the land will eat curds and honey.
>
> Isaiah 7:14,15,21,22

Dairy products can be an excellent, easily utilized form of protein, complementing vegetarian dishes. They are rich sources of calcium, vitamins A, D, E, K, and the B-vitamins, especially riboflavin. Some peoples with limited food variety have thrived on milk products and lived long, vigorous lives. Yet millions of Americans have difficulty with dairy products. What are the reasons and what are our options?

Health Problems

Milk is the number-one allergen in the United States. Many persons are also lactose intolerant, especially those whose ancestral background did not include dairy products. Their bodies do not produce enough of the enzyme lactase to properly digest the lactose (milk sugar) in milk products. The enzyme seems to decrease toward adulthood in many people.

Some nutritionists believe that milk is only for babies and remind us that no animal drinks milk past the weaning stage. Certainly most of us do well to reduce the amount of dairy products we use to cut fat and to make more room for fresh vegetables, fruits, grains, beans, nuts, and seeds in our diets.

For some persons dairy products may cause mucous formation that contributes to congestion, poor digestion, colds, infections, and poor assimilation of nutrients.

Dairy products, as with meats, poultry, and fish, ". . . now contain antibiotics, hormones, pesticides, radioactive isotopes, and other toxic materials—as well as, on occasion, disease-producing bacteria."[1]

Pasteurized Milk

The various forms of dairy products can also make a nutritional difference. Almost all milk is pasteurized. Pasteurization destroys about 38% of the vitamin B-complex, lowers vitamin B_{12} by 12%, destroys the vitamins A and C, reduces the availability of calcium by 10%, lowers protein digestibility by 4% and protein biological value by 17%, and destroys the digestive enzyme phosphatase.[2] Who knows what other unknown nutrient values are reduced or destroyed by pasteurization. Careful studies on animals all reveal better growth and health when raw milk is given. One such study performed on cats by Frances M. Pottenger, Jr., M.D. showed that cats fed pasteurized milk and cooked meat could not reproduce after the second generation. The cats on raw milk and raw meat did not develop this problem.[3] "Pasteurized milk was also tested against raw milk at the West of Scotland Agricultural College, by feeding them to comparable groups of calves. All the calves using the raw milk completed the test period satisfactorily. Those receiving only pasteurized milk became sick or died."[4]

The alternative to pasteurized milk is raw milk. Only raw certified milk (e.g. produced by Alta-Dena Dairy) is sufficiently safe raw milk, however. It is very unfortunate that it has limited availability, primarily to Southern California. The controversy over the safety of raw certified milk is very confusing. Raw certified milk is the only food product in the entire United States that undergoes testing for salmonella bacteria. There are millions of cases of salmonella illness from foods yearly, but Alta-Dena Dairy reports that in 13 years from 1971 through 1983 not one documented illness was ever traced to raw certified dairy products,[5] nor has there been a documented case at any time. In contrast, there have been many thousands of documented cases of illness traced directly to pasteurized milk in various parts of the country with some of the largest outbreaks in the 1980's. Pasteurization does not guarantee the safety of milk as effectively as the high cleanliness standards applied to raw certified milk.

Alta-Dena Dairy has the reputation of being the cleanest dairy in the United States. It was established by the Harold Steuve family with a vision for higher dairy standards to produce a safer milk supply. Alta-Dena Dairy has become a political target because its standards are a threat to the dairy industry that uses pasteurization to compensate for poor standards of cleanliness. Alta-Dena maintains the same high standards of cleanliness for its pasteurized milk as well. Why do not other dairies follow suit? They do not, for the same reason that the tobacco industry does not voluntarily put warning labels on tobacco and cigarettes, and for the same reason that the automobile industry balks at installing safety restraints in cars.

Media reports seldom distinguish between raw milk that is not certified and raw certified milk when discussing the dangers of raw milk. There is risk in consuming any food product. Statistically both our meat and poultry supply and pasteurized milk have proven to be less safe than raw certified milk. We regret that many of our readers cannot enjoy the freedom of choosing the benefits of raw certified milk.

Homogenized Milk

A discussion about raw certified milk is important even if our readers cannot obtain it, because most pasteurized milk is also homogenized. There may be serious problems with homogenized milk as well. The fat molecules in homogenized milk have been altered to keep the fat from rising to the top.

This prolongs shelf life of the milk. *The XO Factor** by Kurt A. Oster, M.D., and Donald J. Ross, Ph.D., details and documents 40 years of research concerning the enzyme, xanthine oxidase, present in cow's milk. Their research shows that a significant amount of xanthine oxidase gets into the bloodstream with the smaller fat molecules of homogenized milk and damages the arterial walls. In turn, the body draws cholesterol, calcium, and other protective agents from the bloodstream to repair the damaged walls. Researchers admit openly that they do not know the cause of initial damage to artery walls that triggers the process of cholesterol deposits. "Scientists are not yet certain why high levels of cholesterol lead to heart disease or what sets the insidious process in motion. The most widely accepted explanation is the so-called injury theory, propounded by Russell Ross at the University of Washington in Seattle. According to Ross, 'the disease begins with damage to the thin layer of cells, or endothelium, that forms the protective lining of the arteries.' "[6] Perhaps there are several causes from our faulty diet. Could xanthine oxidase be one of them?

It is unfortunate that the scientific community has not yet seen fit to set aside vested interests and objectively investigate this theory. A historical lesson may remind us not to place total confidence upon orthodox views. In the nineteenth century Ignaz Semmelweis discovered that women died in childbirth because disease was carried in hospitals from person to person with doctors' unwashed hands. Semmelweis developed a method of hand washing that saved many lives. Yet his theory was not only rejected, he was also dismissed from his hospital position, and the antiseptic method of cleansing hands and instruments was not officially introduced until over 30 years later. It was not until 1960 that a

---

*Homogenized! by Nicolas Sampsidis, M.S., presents a shorter and easy to read account of Oster's and Ross's work.

book describing a method of washing the hands approximating the biblical method in Numbers 19 was written by the New York State Department of Health following a staph infection epidemic in 1958 caused by improperly washed hands.[7] While we wait for the scientific community to respond to the research regarding xanthine oxidase, we suggest caution in using homogenized milk as a dietary mainstay for our children.

Milk Choices

What are our options? Our first option is whole milk. Whole milk may provide too much fat for many people. Yet when the fat is removed so are most of the fat-soluble vitamins A, D, E, and K. Although vitamins A and D are synthetically restored to skim or nonfat milk, we wonder how well this fortification matches the original nutrient value. Lowfat milk is a compromise between skim or nonfat and whole milk. What form of whole, lowfat, or nonfat milk is best?

Goat's milk is a wonderful choice because it is closer in composition to human milk than cow's milk. If you have access to it and it fits into your food budget, by all means take advantage of it. We have chosen to use Alta-Dena or Stueve's Natural raw certified milk products because they are available to us. We make our own lowfat milk by blending equal amounts of raw certified whole milk and nonfat milk. We also use raw certified butter, buttermilk, cottage cheese, kefir, jack cheese, and cheddar cheeses. Some of these latter raw certified products are available in many states throughout the U.S.A.

If raw certified milk is unavailable, we recommend nonfat or skim milk. It may be fortified by blending in nonfat dry milk powder from the health food store or instant nonfat dry milk from the supermarket. Add at least 1/3 cup per quart of nonfat milk, allowing it to refrigerate several hours to improve flavor. Nonfat dry milk can also be added freely to fortify baked goods. Use it as a replacement for half the sugar taken out of a recipe when honey is used. Keep in mind that nonfat milk will not provide original fat-soluble vitamins. Therefore, be certain to also include plenty of whole grains, and dark green and yellow vegetables in the menu.

If homogenized milk is used, xanthine oxidase can be inactivated by simmering at 195° F. for 10 to 15 seconds. This will alter the taste.

If you have a milk sugar (lactose) intolerance, inquire of your doctor, a nutritionist, or your local health food store for new products that assist the body to digest it better. Digestive enzyme preparations, Lactaid™ or Lactase™, are available at drugstores without prescription.

Cultured Milks

Cultured milks include yogurt, kefir, and buttermilk. When raw certified milk is not available, cultured milks are perhaps the best alternative available. They are easier to digest because part of the milk lactose has been converted to lactic acid. Even some persons allergic to sweet milk can tolerate some form of cultured milk. Yogurt and kefir contain live bacteria cultures that help the body to produce its own friendly bacteria in the colon to fight toxic bacteria and to produce its own B-vitamins. Not all yogurt is prepared with live bacteria. Any yogurt labeled with only gelatin added is not made with live bacteria. Yogurt with live bacteria will be labeled viable cultures, live bacteria, lactobacillus acidophilus, or acidophilus cultures. Also, we recommend yogurt not sweetened with refined sugars. Nonfat and lowfat yogurts are best. No raw certified yogurt is commercially available.

Cheeses

Cheese is an excellent food, but hard cheeses are very high in fat except for a few. Mozzarella cheese is the best known and most widely available. It contains half the fat content of cheddar cheeses. We prefer cheeses that do not have food coloring added. If the cheese is yellow, coloring has been added. Use natural cheddar cheeses in preference to processed American cheeses. Small amounts of Parmesan and Romano cheeses are good choices, especially freshly grated. Both ricotta and lowfat cottage cheese are lower in fat than hard cheeses. All cheeses have quite a bit of sodium in them unless otherwise labeled "low" or "no" sodium.

What About Calcium?

If you do not use dairy products, sufficient calcium may be obtained in other ways, although not as easily from other foods. Check the Best Food Sources for Vitamins and Minerals list (p. 101) for other high-calcium food sources. A calcium supplement such as bone meal, calcium gluconate, or calcium lactate can be easily added to the diet. The amount of calcium available to the body is also influenced by other food habits. Excessive protein and refined sugars, for example, draw calcium from the body. Again many things work together for or against health.

Conclusion

Weston A. Price, D.D.S., reports in his book, *Nutrition And Physical Degeneration*: "The most physically perfect people in northern India are probably the Pathans who live on dairy products largely in the form of soured curd, together with wheat and vegetables."[8] Perhaps many of the problems of eating dairy products have more to do with what modern food technology has done to them. According to the Eating Better Lifestyle Chart (p. 29) you can see that the emphasis of our diet is not placed on dairy products in the forms available to us in the U.S.A.

Summary of Dairy Product Choices:

Milk:

1st choice: goat's milk
cultured dairy products (raw certified,
if possible) such as
nonfat or lowfat yogurts,
kefir, buttermilk

2nd choice: lowfat or nonfat milk (raw
certified, if possible) such as
pasteurized nonfat or lowfat
yogurts, kefir, buttermilk

With caution: yogurts prepared with homogenized
whole milk

Avoid: homogenized milk

Cheeses:

1st choice: raw certified natural cheeses with no
food coloring
mozzarella cheese
Parmesan and Romano cheese
(fresh whole)
lowfat cottage cheese (raw
certified, if possible)
ricotta cheese
low sodium types

2nd choice: natural cheddar cheeses (pasteurized)
Parmesan and Romano cheeses (grated)

Avoid: processed cheeses and cheese foods

Cooking Recommendation: Heat milk as little as possible. Bring just to a boil when necessary. Use cultured milks (buttermilk, yogurt) in preference to sweet milk in baking.

Emilie's Cheese Storage Hints:

Soft, ripened cheeses such as brie and camembert freeze well; wrap tightly. It is best to freeze whole wheels or large pieces. Semi-hard and hard cheeses such as cheddar will slice poorly and will crumble once frozen.

Two cubes of sugar stored with any cheese in an air-tight container will help to retard the growth of mold.

All cheeses are more flavorful at room temperature than when cold. However, hard cheeses are easier to slice while still cold.

22

Those Magnificent Micronutrients

> I will give you the treasures of darkness, riches
> stored in secret places, so that you may know that I
> am the LORD.
>
> Isaiah 45:3

Vitamins interact in thousands of ways with enzymes to carry on all body processes, while minerals are an integral part of all body tissue and involved in many body processes as well. Each vitamin and mineral performs so many life-giving functions that they are truly a great wonder of our Lord's creative genius and power! We cannot possibly list the many tasks of the micronutrients in such a short space. The *Nutrition Almanac* is an excellent reference on vitamins and minerals.

The fact that the first vitamin was not discovered until as recently as 1886 ought to arouse skepticism about the completeness of synthetic vitamins, either in tablet form or in refined foods fortified with them. Persons who insist that the body does not know the difference between synthetic and natural vitamins overlook the probability of unknown nutrients contained in the natural forms. Whole foods will best supply what is yet undiscovered.

Prevention of deficiency diseases such as beriberi, pellagra, anemia, or scurvy is not a good measure of adequate vitamin and mineral intake. It is this view that fostered the enrichment of white flour with vitamins B_1, B_2, B_3, and iron. We now know that the complete range of micronutrients is vital in our resistance to illnesses, degenerative diseases, and premature aging. Americans by the millions are suffering marginal vitamin and mineral deficiencies fostered by the refined food diet. For example, the loss of vitamin E in white flour is 86%, yet vitamin E plays a key role in the prevention of heart disease. The implication is that millions suffer from heart disease not only because of high fat intake but also from vitamin E deficiency. This means that our supply of vitamins and minerals in whole foods is just as vital to health and disease prevention as low fat and high fiber.

The only way to guarantee the complete micronutrient package is to eat a varied diet of whole foods. It is not necessary or practical to count micrograms or milligrams of vitamins and minerals to make sure you are getting enough. A varied diet of whole foods that provides enough calories, protein, carbohydrates, and fat will usually provide all the vitamins and minerals you can get from food. While many persons in America may also need to support the diet with additional vitamin and mineral supplements, all need the foundation of the Eating Better Lifestyle.

The Best Food Sources for Vitamins and Minerals list begins on page 101. This will guide you in choosing the variety of foods that supply them. Keep in mind that vitamins and minerals are widely distributed throughout all foods. You will receive small amounts from many varied food sources. Water-soluble vitamins, the B-vitamins and vitamin C, are washed out of the body daily and, therefore, must be replenished daily. Fat-soluble vitamins and minerals can be stored in the body. It is almost impossible to get an overdose of any vitamin or mineral from eating a variety of whole foods.

Vitamin A in animal foods and plant foods is not the same. Plant foods contain carotene, or provitamin A. The human body manufactures vitamin A out of carotene, utilizing only $1/4$ to $1/2$ the carotene in plant foods. This means that 10,000 to 20,000 International Units (I.U.'s) of carotene must be eaten to produce 5,000 I.U.'s of vitamin A in the body. The body will utilize about half the carotene from leafy green vegetables and about a fourth from root vegetables such as carrots.

Proper food storage and preparation will affect the availability of vitamins and minerals. In general, vitamin C and the B-vitamins are the most perishable, easily destroyed by air, heat, and light. To preserve vitamin C and other nutrients, store all foods except those with protective skins in tightly covered containers. Store fresh foods away from light in the refrigerator or in cold storage. Do not leave them at room temperature long before preparation and eating. Cover fruits that are cut longer than ten minutes before serving or turn the cut side toward the plate. Eat many fruits and vegetables raw. Cook vegetables lightly, just until crisp-tender. Quick stir-fry or steaming will preserve vegetable nutrients the best. If you boil them in water, use only a very small amount. The exception is broccoli (p. 264). Save the cooking water to use in soups, breads, and bean or grain dishes. Keep a covered jar handy to store leftover vegetable water in the refrigerator.

An excellent reference to whole food storage is *Keeping Food Fresh* by Janet Bailey.

Best Food Sources of Vitamins and Minerals

Vitamin A (fat soluble)
o.g.* liver of beef, lamb, poultry, cheeses, eggs, whole milk, halibut, mackerel, fish liver oil

Provitamin A (carotene) (fat soluble)
vegetables: all dark leafy greens (spinach, kale, beet greens, collards, chard, mustard greens, sorrel, turnip greens, dandelion greens, lamb's-quarters), dark yellow vegetables (carrots, sweet potatoes, yams [U.S. variety], yellow squash, pumpkin), broccoli, endive, arugula, loose-leaf lettuce, romaine lettuce, red peppers, tomatoes, parsley, ruta-bagas, brussels sprouts, green beans, asparagus, lima beans, green peas, sweet corn
fruits: apricots, cantaloupe, sour cherries, mango, nec-tarine, papaya, peach, persimmon, watermelon

Vitamin C (water soluble)
vegetables: dark leafy greens (collards, kale, spinach, mus-tard greens, turnip greens, sorrel, lamb's-quarters), broc-coli, cabbage, green and red peppers, okra, green peas, brussels sprouts, parsley, Irish potatoes, sweet potatoes, yams (U.S. variety), cauliflower, tomatoes
fruits: citrus (orange, grapefruit, tangerine, lemon, lime), kiwi fruit, pineapple, papaya, mango, berries (strawberries, loganberries, blackberries, raspberries), guava, honeydew melon, cantaloupe

Vitamin D (fat soluble)
fish liver oil (cod, halibut), sardines, herring, salmon, tuna, egg yolks, fortified milk

Vitamin E (fat soluble)
whole grains, vegetable oils (unrefined or cold-pressed safflower, soybean, corn), soybeans, eggs, dark leafy greens,

---

*Organically grown. Liver can be very toxic if not organically grown. For definition of organically grown, see p. 143.

broccoli, brussels sprouts, cabbage, asparagus, raw nuts and seeds, peanuts

Vitamin K (fat soluble)
yogurt, egg yolks, beef, blackstrap molasses, vegetable oils (sunflower, safflower, soybean), fish liver oils, kelp, leafy green vegetables (cabbage, kale, spinach), green peas, carrots, cauliflower, tomatoes—and the human body can make vitamin K

Vitamin P (Biflavonoids or C Complex) (water soluble)
white skins of citrus fruits, apricots, buckwheat, green peppers, tomatoes, apricots, rhubarb, blackberries, cherries, rose hips

Essential Fatty Acids (Linoleic, Linolenic, Arachidonic)
vegetable oils (sunflower, safflower, soybean, peanut), wheat germ in whole wheat, sunflower seeds, walnuts, pecans, almonds, avocados—and the human body can make linolenic and arachidonic (if enough linoleic is present)

B-Vitamins (water soluble)
B-vitamins generally are present together in the same foods; whole grains, eggs, leafy greens

B_1 *(Thiamine)*
whole grains, peanuts, beef kidney, milk, eggs, plums, prunes, raisins, blackstrap molasses

B_2 *(Riboflavin)*
milk; o.g. liver, kidney, and heart of lamb, beef, veal; cheese, green vegetables, broccoli, eggs

B_3 *(Niacin)*
whole grains; o.g. liver of beef, chicken, veal, and lamb; eggs, lean meat, poultry, fish (swordfish, tuna, halibut), roasted peanuts, dates, figs, avocados, prunes—and the human body can make niacin

B_6 *(Pyridoxine)*
whole rye flour, brown rice, buckwheat (kasha), whole

wheat; o.g. liver and heart; chicken, beef, eggs, cantaloupe, cabbage, blackstrap molasses, fish (herring,
mackerel, salmon), peanuts, soybeans, walnuts

B_{12} (Cobalamin)
milk; o.g. liver of lamb, beef; veal, egg yolks, fish (herring, salmon, sardines)

B_{13} (Orotic acid)
whey (cultured dairy), root vegetables

B_{15} (Pangamic Acid)
whole grains, brown rice, pumpkin seeds, sesame seeds,
o.g. liver

B_{17} (laetrile) (amygdalin)
whole grains, legumes (dry beans), wild berries, kernels
of apricots, apples, cherries, peaches, plums, nectarines,
cashews, macadamia nuts, sprouts (alfalfa, mung, garbanzo, wheat), unhulled sesame seeds, flax seeds, chia
seeds

Biotin
wheat, milk, o.g. beef liver, egg yolks, chicken, salmon,
brown rice, nuts, fruits, corn, mushrooms—and the
human body can make biotin

Pantothenic Acid
wheat, eggs; o.g. liver, kidney and heart of beef, chicken,
and lamb; green vegetables, herring, whole grains, nuts,
raw peanuts

Choline
wheat; o.g. beef liver, heart, and brain; leafy green vegetables, peanuts

Folic Acid
whole wheat, dark leafy greens, egg yolks; o.g. liver of
beef, lamb, and chicken; tuna, cantaloupe, asparagus,
carrots, apricots, pumpkins, avocados, beans, dark rye
flour

Inositol
> whole wheat; o.g. beef heart, liver, and brain; cantaloupe, cabbage, raisins, dried limas, grapefruit—and the human body can make inositol

PABA (Para-aminobenzoic Acid)
> whole grains, brown rice, liver, kidney, molasses, yogurt—and the human body can make PABA

Calcium
> milk, cheeses, cottage cheese, yogurt, sardines, salmon, cooked leafy green vegetables (beet greens, spoon cabbage, chard, kale, collards, mustard greens, turnip greens, dandelion greens, lamb's-quarters), broccoli, okra, dried beans, unhulled sesame seeds, blackstrap molasses, carob, rhubarb

Chlorine
> salt, kelp, dulse, plant seafood, rye flour, ripe olives

Chromium
> meat, chicken, corn oil, brewer's yeast (supplement)

Cobalt
> meat, kidney, liver, milk, plant seafood

Copper
> leafy green vegetables, dried beans, peas, whole grains, prunes, almonds, most seafood, calf and beef liver

Fluorine
> seafoods, gelatin

Iodine
> kelp, onions, plant seafood, fish, vegetables grown in iodine-rich soil (especially mushrooms)

Iron
> beef liver, heart, kidney; lean red meat, dried peaches, egg yolks, nuts, beans, asparagus, blackstrap molasses, oatmeal, leafy green vegetables

Magnesium
figs, lemons, grapefruit, apples, green vegetables, yellow corn, soybeans, wheat, almonds, nuts, seeds

Manganese
leafy green vegetables, peas, beets, nuts, whole grains, egg yolks

Molybdenum
dark leafy green vegetables, whole grains, legumes

Phosphorus
fish, poultry, meat, whole grains, eggs, nuts, seeds

Potassium
citrus fruits, watercress, all green leafy vegetables, mint leaves, sunflower seeds, bananas, potatoes (especially peelings), oranges, whole grains

Selenium
whole wheat, tuna fish, onions, broccoli, tomatoes

Sodium
salt, carrots, beets, artichokes, kelp, seafoods, poultry, meat

Sulfur
brussels sprouts, cabbage, dried beans, nuts, eggs, fish, lean beef

Vanadium
fish

Zinc
whole grains, eggs, ground mustard, round steak, lamb chops, pumpkin seeds, brewer's yeast (supplement)

23

The Sensation of Sugar

> Eat honey, my son, for it is good. . . . If you find
> honey, eat just enough. . . . It is not good to eat too
> much honey. . . .
>
> Proverbs 24:13; 25:16,27

Why do we seek out sweet foods? When man gathered
foods from the wild, sweet plants were usually safe in contrast to the bitter which were often poisonous. It was probably
man's instinct for the sweet taste that led him to seek out
sweet fruits containing choice nutrients such as vitamin C
and natural quick-energy-producing sugars. It is not our
inherited drive for sweet things that is at fault. It is the many
refined food products that retain the sweetness but not the
nutrients. Food companies know that we love them and,
therefore, spend $400 million yearly to advertise foods on
television. Half of them are sugary foods.

Sugar was first cultivated in India in 325 B.C., but remained
a scarce luxury for many centuries. It became a common food
only in the last 100 years. Today the average sugar consumption yearly in America is 125 pounds or 600 calories per day,[1]
at least 24% of the total diet, consumed primarily through
thousands of prepackaged foods. Only 3% of calories come
from fruits and vegetables and 3% from milk. Despite all the
publicity that we need to cut sugar intake, Americans are
gobbling it up more than ever. The big food companies are
getting rich on our inherent desire for sweets!

Why is it so important to cut sugar intake and to choose
nutritious sources? Dr. Ray C. Wunderlich, Jr., M.D. in his
book *Sugar and Your Health* summarizes for us: "Although
refined sugar is not the cause of all health problems, it comes
closer to qualifying for that position than most other single
factors."[2]

Not all will agree that refined sugar is death in the pot, yet its effects on health have been extensively researched. Sugar has been implicated in the following effects on bodily health:

—Increased blood cholesterol and triglyceride levels that contribute to heart disease

—Unstable blood sugar levels that contribute to hypoglycemia, diabetes, and aggravate criminal behavior

—Depletion of B-vitamins stored in the body which contributes to depression, an intensified craving for alcohol in alcoholics, and excessive estrogen in women that contributes to breast cancer[3]

—Displacement of more nutritious foods with empty calories contributing to obesity, and lowered resistance to most health problems and degenerative diseases

—Upset of the homeostasis (balance) mechanism which causes a perpetual craving for sugar—sugar addiction

—Increased uric acid in the blood leading to gout

—Reduction of phosphorus in the blood that prevents bone calcification, and leaching of calcium from the bones that contributes to osteoporosis

—Altered pH (acid/base) balance in the mouth which causes tooth decay

—Reduced effectiveness of white blood cells to kill bacteria, thus encouraging infections

What are some ways to reduce refined sugar consumption? What are the alternatives? If we lived on a sugar plantation, we could chew on sugar cane, a whole food nutrient package. Chewing on sugar cane is not the same as consuming white sugar from which all the original fiber and nutrients are extracted. Fresh fruits, our best sources of natural sweets, are widely available. They are truly God's desserts requiring little or no preparation. Nevertheless, most of us want some sweetening to cook with, too. What is the best?

There is only one sugar that is not manufactured—honey. The biblical record for honey sets aside the argument that honey is no better than refined sugar. God's Word is especially clear about this particular food: "Eat honey, my son, for it is good . . . but not too much." We wonder if God had the twentieth century in mind! He created honey as a whole, natural food with a wealth of nutritional value, minute as the amounts may be. Arguments that these amounts are too small to count are presumptuous. Besides, God gave the Israelites "a land flowing with milk and honey." Would He expect them not to eat the honey? Its goodness is extolled by those who have learned to appreciate it:

> Containing 39 percent fructose, honey is an important antifatigue food. Since it is predigested, it builds up alkaline reserves in the blood and tissues, and provides a maximum of energy with a minimum of shock to the digestive system. Sugar-laden foods overload the bloodstream in 15 minutes; honey is absorbed over a period of four hours.

> There is no energy-producing food on the market to touch honey. Nor will there ever be. All synthetic glucose products are inferior to honey, not only for the speed with which they bring about a sense of well-being, but also for the production of real lasting energy and the alkalinizing of the body.[4]

Honey contains minute amounts of a wealth of nutrients including B-vitamins, vitamin C, and at least 12 minerals. It has many other nutrient properties not fully understood, including bee pollen protein of high value. Honey is easily and rapidly assimilated, provides a natural, gentle laxative effect, and is easier on the kidneys to process than all other sugars. The nutrients in honey assist in its partial digestion. When combined with whole grain flour or cereal high in dietary fiber and B-vitamins, the body can digest honey very well without depleting stored nutrients in the body.

We must also heed the biblical warning not to eat too much honey. Start by reducing the number of desserts and sweets.

Sugar intake can be reduced further by using half as much honey as white sugar in recipes, since it is twice as sweet. The strong flavor curbs appetite, too. The flavor depends on what flowers the bees visited to collect nectar. Lighter honey is usually a milder flavor. You may prefer a milder honey for puddings and toppings, but a darker honey works well in baking. Like olive oil, honey is an expensive ingredient. This hidden blessing will also limit our use of it!

As with other good foods, honey can be refined. Heating over 160° and straining removes valuable bee pollen and some of the nutrients. Supermarket honey and much of it in health food stores is refined. The best quality honey is unheated, unfiltered honey. Honey labeled "uncooked" does not classify as "unheated," because it can be heated to 160° and still be labeled "uncooked." Top-quality honey is a very expensive health food store item. Purchasing honey in five-gallon cans from a local beekeeper will be the least expensive. Honey can be stored indefinitely. If supermarket honey is the only honey available to you, use it as a first step to breaking the refined sugar habit.

Since heating honey destroys some of its nutritional value, heat it as little as possible when cooking over direct heat, adding it toward the last of the cooking process. When honey is used in baking, it is protected somewhat by being combined with other ingredients.

Although honey is our first choice, there are other alternatives to white sugar. These include pure maple syrup, blackstrap molasses, sorghum, date sugar, and granulated fructose. All of these are expensive and not as widely available as honey. The health food store is the best place to find them. Pure maple syrup has a good amount of potassium and calcium. Don't confuse it with supermarket pancake syrup that is made with white sugar or corn syrup and imitation maple flavoring. Pure maple syrup comes from maple trees. Use it occasionally for pancakes and waffles. Sorghum is high in calcium, phosphorus, riboflavin, niacin, and iron. Blackstrap molasses contains most of the nutrients refined out of white sugar. It is high in calcium, potassium, and iron. It has a stronger flavor and more nutrient value than the light and dark molasses sold in supermarkets. Date sugar, actually ground dates, is high in potassium, B-vitamins, and vitamin A. Granulated fructose, derived primarily from corn, contains little nutrient value. Its two advantages over white sugar are that it requires less release of insulin in the body and, like honey, it is twice as sweet as sugar, requiring half the amount in recipes. We use it only in an occasional recipe, such as angel food cake, where honey really does not work very well.

All of these sugars are combinations of the simple sugars—fructose, glucose, maltose, and sucrose. Fresh fruits, fruit juices, high fructose corn syrup, and honey are highest in fructose. Maltose is the form of sugar primarily in milk and beer. Molasses, white and brown sugar, maple syrup, raw and turbinado sugar, and sorghum are all primarily sucrose. Refined sugars used in prepackaged foods include high fructose corn syrup, corn syrup solids, dextrose, dextrins, invert sugar, sucrose, and glucose. A most effective way to remove refined sugars from the diet is to replace prepackaged foods with basic whole foods. In addition there are some prepacked foods in health food stores that do not contain refined sugars.

What about artificial sweeteners such as saccharin, cyclamates, Equal, NutraSweet, and aspartame? The history of saccharin and cyclamates should suggest to us that the current unchecked use of aspartame in hundreds of food products is not a guaranteed measure of its boon to health. Aspartame, also known as Equal and NutraSweet, has been pronounced safe by the Federal Food and Drug Administration. The FDA has undoubtedly been pressured by large food businesses that wish to use aspartame in many products. In the meantime many news articles have appeared that report concern about the effects of aspartame, especially in regard to brain chemistry. Problematic effects from aspartame seem most likely to occur when several cans of soda pop with aspartame are consumed with carbohydrates such as a sandwich or a candy bar. There is also some concern that aspartame may adversely affect the unborn baby. We do not have sufficient information about aspartame to make a wise judgment. We suggest caution in using Equal, or food products containing aspartame and NutraSweet, and that pregnant women avoid them altogether. Finally, we may ask the question, "Can man develop any imitation food that equals the nutritional life-giving value of God's original whole foods?"

What is the sugarholic to do? There is hope! If you are addicted to sugar, there are several things you can do to break the habit. A frequent protein snack such as an egg, piece of cheese, or plain yogurt may help. Protein can curb a sugar craving by stablizing the blood sugar level. Eating several small snacks throughout the day of fresh fruit, nuts, seeds, or raw vegetables can help. All of these contain natural sugars that will produce a slow rise in blood sugar level. Many people are especially helped by eating nuts and seeds. Try unsalted and unroasted sunflower seeds. They are least expensive. Soaking sunflower seeds or almonds in water for 2 to 8 hours before eating them will improve digestibility. Soaked sunflower seeds have a very pleasing crunch. Nuts and seeds must be chewed very well to digest properly. Blending a few of them in protein shakes will help, too. An increase in unrefined complex carbohydrate foods that are high in B-vitamins such as breads and cereals also will decrease the sugar craving. You may be able to enjoy eating whole grain muffins* in place of sugary foods. Try them. The honey content is much lower than in cakes, cookies, and desserts. Remove all the refined sugars from the house. A fast for up to three days, especially with prayer, can break a food craving. Exercise will also add to your arsenal of weapons against the craving for sugar.

---

*For muffin recipes information see p. 287.

Cooking with Honey Tip: Reduce oven temperature by 25° when substituting honey for white or brown sugar in any favorite recipe.

Honey for Babies? Wait until baby has passed the first birthday before feeding honey. Botulism spores may be in honey and are potentially dangerous for infants under one year. There is no known danger to anyone older. Furthermore, there is no point in introducing any kind of concentrated sugar to a baby.

Emilie's Beauty Aid: I clean my face, then put honey all over my face and relax 10-15 minutes—rinse well. Smooth, soft skin appears.

24

Raw Foods in Review

> On each side of the river stood the tree of life, bearing twelve crops of fruit, yielding its fruit every month. And the leaves of the tree are for the healing of the nations.
>
> Revelation 22:2

The Eating Better Lifestyle includes lots of fresh fruits and vegetables. No vitamins and minerals are lost in cooking. Their high content of pure water assists in cleansing waste products from the body. Chlorophyll in green plants is also very cleansing for the bloodstream.

Nutritionists do not agree on the benefit of plant enzymes to the human body, but many believe that they are vital to human health. Some even claim that raw foods are the only kind that mankind should eat because all enzymes are destroyed by cooking. Whether or not our bodies need the enzymes, raw foods have enough advantages to warrant a favored place in our diet.

It is unlikely that many Americans would adopt an all-raw-foods diet on a long-term basis, but a short-term diet of all raw food for a week or two can help to rejuvenate the body. It might be good to know that if you lose your cooking facilities or fuel, you can thrive on raw foods. You can also sprout seeds, grains, and beans. Vitamins and minerals are multiplied many times from the original seed, bean, or grain when grown into sprouts. The protein value of sprouts is also excellent.

It is easy to grow alfalfa sprouts. Soak 2 tablespoons of alfalfa seeds from a health food store in a quart jar covered with a piece of screen held in place with a rubber band. Soak overnight, drain, and tip the jar downward in a bowl on your kitchen counter. Water the sprouts once every morning and evening keeping them well drained. In five to seven days your jar will be full of fresh sprouts to use in sandwiches and salads or to snack on. Cover them tightly and refrigerate. They will keep up to two weeks. For the value of their nutrition, sprouts are the most inexpensive food. They are also free of pesticides.

There is nothing like vine-ripened fresh produce for nutrition and flavor. Garden growing provides a wonderful opportunity and is often our only chance to get fresh food grown without pesticides. Eat the peelings on fruits and vegetables as much as possible because much of the nutrient content is near the surface. Scrub fresh produce well. Leafy greens may have been sprayed with pesticide as many as eight times. Fill the sink with water and add 2 tablespoons of apple cider vinegar. Immerse vegetables such as the leafy greens, broccoli, brussels sprouts, and parsley. Do this two or more times and rinse thoroughly. Spin the water out of leafy greens. Add a paper towel inside the storage bag to soak up excess moisture.

Avoid buying potatoes that have a greenish tinge. The discoloration is caused by prolonged exposure to light, developing a toxic poison called solanine and giving the potatoes a slightly bitter taste. If you must use such potatoes, peel them and trim away all the green part. Store potatoes properly in a dark, humid, well-ventilated place at a cool 45-50°. You can store them in the refrigerator if needed.

Recycle your produce scraps in the compost pile outside in the garden area. Your garbage disposal doesn't need them!

25

A Salty Sermon

Salt is good. . . .   Luke 14:34

Is tasteless food eaten without salt . . .? I refuse
to touch it; such food makes me ill.

Job 6:6,7

The American Diet averages 10,000 to 20,000 milligrams of sodium per day. The Recommended Dietary Allowance is 1,100 to 3,300 milligrams per day. The Eating Better Lifestyle menus and recipes allow you to use salt in cooking and baking, yet within the 1,100 to 3,300 milligram range.* Below this range, taste becomes an obstacle to many people. Actually the human body requires only 500 milligrams or less of sodium per day which can be obtained from our food without the addition of salt. Learning to season food well without salt requires skill and practice. The following guidelines will help to curb the sodium level without eliminating salt altogether:

—Leave salt off the table.
—Do not salt vegetables while cooking.
—Save the salt for baking and main dishes or other flavorful recipes such as soups. Season to taste to reduce original amount called for.
—Use low-sodium baking powder in baking (available at health food stores).

---

*The "no salt" diet is a therapeutic diet (see p. 42). The Eating Better Lifestyle is not a therapeutic diet, although recipes and menus are adaptable with specific modifications.

With the freedom to use a little salt, the taste of whole foods—especially grains and beans—will go from bland to delightful.

Purchase a higher-quality salt with trace minerals and containing neither aluminum nor dextrose which has not been kiln dried. Most of these salts are labeled as sea salt, but not all sea salts are of the same quality. Look for the label "sun evaporated only," or for "unheated" salt. (See p. 218 for a mail order resource.)

A reduction from 10,000 mg. or more of sodium in the diet to 3,300 mg. or less is a great improvement and quite adequate for most people. In order to do this, of course, you will need to omit packaged foods with salt added. But do not be overly concerned about using canned tomato products or tuna fish unless you make dishes with them every day. They are both very high in sodium, but you can still use some in cooking. Tomato paste is much lower than tomato sauce in sodium. We are also finding canned tomatoes on the supermarket shelves with no salt, so check the labels carefully. Lemon juice added to unsalted tuna compensates for the lack of salt.

High blood pressure is a serious problem. Sixty million persons have it, and many do not even know it. It is the leading cause of strokes and the cause of about 30% of all heart disease. In addition many overweight persons have a water retention problem. Salt consumption, however, is not the sole cause of high blood pressure and water retention. The lack of calcium in the diet along with accompanying low levels of potassium, vitamin A, and vitamin C may have just as much or more to do with these problems. David A. McCarron, M.D., in *Science* (June 29, 1984) reported the findings of a study involving calcium and high blood pressure. "We've always thought of heart disease in terms of excesses, especially excesses of sodium and cholesterol, . . . But these patterns are patterns of deficiency . . . so let's deal with these deficiencies and step back from hammering on dietary restrictions. "[1] This study also demonstrated a correlation between higher consumption of dairy products and lower blood pressure levels. "Increased consumption of dairy products would be associated with a correction in potassium and calcium deficits."[2] Dr. McCarron states that if we consumed at least 800 milligrams of calcium daily (the RDA for the average adult) and 3,000 to 3,500 milligrams of potassium, "It's likely that sodium will take care of itself."[3] There is evidence that magnesium levels are also involved. Denise Foley reports in "Foods to Lower Your Blood Pressure," *Prevention* (July, 1984, p. 30), ". . . one of the most interesting things to come out of Dr. McCarron's research is not how calcium works alone to lower blood pressure but how it works with potassium, sodium and magnesium to regulate pressure. 'It's the proportions of these minerals in the body that seem to be the most important thing,' says Dr. McCarron." Again we are talking about synergism (things working best in combination) and that is just what a diet of whole food variety provides! We believe this is more important than omitting all salt from cooking.

Small amounts of potassium, calcium, and magnesium are widely distributed in whole foods, but some are especially good sources. The chart on page 101 will guide you in choosing these foods. Other findings point to EPA and DHA (also called omega-3 fatty acids) in fish and linoleic acid in polyunsaturated oils as nutrients that contribute to normal blood pressure. High-fiber foods and exercise are also important for normal blood pressure.

26

I'm Sick and Tired
of Being Fat!

In the last ten years I have gained 30 diet books and lost 200 lbs—the same 10 lbs. over and over and over . . . !

American obsession. People even die from the fear of it. We call that anorexia and bulimia. We still believe that "fatty, fatty, two by four, can't get through the kitchen door," is a social disgrace! We believe it at the cost of every new diet rage that hits the newsstands. No matter if "diets don't work," we'll try them anyway, again, again, and again! Each new diet proclaims the same sensational promise: "It works!" Yet 95% of 34 million overweight people (25% of the American population) continue to experience the truth of Proverbs 13:12, step A: "Hope deferred makes the heart sick . . ." We never achieve the hope of step B: "but a longing fulfilled is a tree of life." Witness the following scenario:

> Begin new diet, lose weight rapidly for two-three-four weeks, hit plateau, get discouraged, hang in there while losing more pounds—more slowly, reach "ideal" weight—hurrah!, return to "normal" diet—hungrier than ever, gain back more pounds than lost on diet! Guilty! "Must not have done it right. Must gain more self-control. It couldn't have been the diet, it must have been me! Maybe I can do better on the next diet."

Stop! It's time to get off this hopeless diet merry-go-round and get on the road of hope and health! How are we going to do that? First we need to understand why low-calorie dieting fails.

Why Diets Don't Work

The historical norm is not perpetual feast, but periodic food shortage and famine. For example, two-thirds of the world population is currently hungry. There are many biblical accounts of famine such as Genesis 12:10, "Now there was a famine in the land, and Abram went down to Egypt to live there for a while because the famine was severe . . ."; Genesis 41:57, "And all the countries came to Egypt to buy grain from Joseph, because the famine was severe in all the world . . ."; Ruth 1:1, "In the days when the judges ruled, there was a famine in the land . . ."; 2 Samuel 21:1, "During the reign of David, there was a famine for three successive years . . ."; 1 Kings 18:2, "Now the famine was severe in Samaria . . ."; Acts 11:28, "One of them, named Agabus, stood up and through the Spirit predicted that a severe famine would spread over the entire Roman world . . . "; Matthew 24:7, "There will be famines and earthquakes in various places."

God designed our bodies to burn fewer calories in times of food shortage and famine to prolong life on slim pickin's. How good of Him! Our hope of winning the war on weight is partially destroyed by low-calorie diets because they create an artificial famine. Therefore, adopting a low-calorie diet makes it very difficult to return to a normal calorie level without gaining even more weight back than was lost.

We see Christians struggling to apply spiritual principles to a discipline of dieting that accomplishes just the opposite of what they work and pray for because they are not aware of the way God designed their bodies. The result adds spiritual, emotional, and mental stress creating volumes of guilt. Our affluence and abundance, an abnormal situation, requires a different approach to weight control than dieting.

Step off the diet merry-go-round and forget about all of those low-calorie diets! What a relief! June Bailey thinks so, too. She has written a book, *Fat Is Where It's At*. Bailey has decided to accept herself as she is. "I've learned to like the fat person who lives in this body."[1] She is on the right track.

Personal Worth Not Measured in Inches 'n Pounds

"Your beauty . . . should be that of your inner self, the unfading beauty of a gentle and quiet spirit, which is of great worth in God's sight. For this is the way the holy women of the past who put their hope in God used to make themselves beautiful" (1 Peter 3:3-5). Our friend Helen, though she struggles with being overweight, is a lovely example. We observed her recently as she demonstrated her professional expertise in producing and directing our video, "Eating Better with Sue." When she is not producing and editing films, she is caring for her lively twin two-year-old boys, caring for her hard-working husband, and leading an Inner Development group. She radiates the love of Christ in her relationships. Her inner beauty comes through her eyes, her smile, her conversation, and her touch, and it is this that dominates her outward appearance. This is the kind of beauty that God looks for. It is the unseen that is eternal. It is not that God is disinterested in one's struggle with obesity. But He does not measure personal worth by it. If this is not your view of yourself, stop now and pray for God's sense of your worth without reference to your body size. As you gain this frame of mind, you can lose your taste for the next fad diet and pursue the Eating Better Lifestyle with a gentle and quiet spirit.

Focus on Total Health

Obesity is seldom, if ever, an isolated health problem. When one focuses on weight loss, calories become more important than the total nutrient value of food. For example, low-calorie diet products and recipes frequently contain ingredients of inferior nutritional quality. In addition, it is not easy to get the full Recommended Dietary Allowances of food nutrients on a 1,500-calorie diet. Success depends on a permanent lifestyle change in eating habits rather than temporary change. Instead of thinking "fewer calories to lose weight," think, "total nutritional value for total health." Helen, for example, has decided to approach eating in this way. The result is a new focus, not upon her own individual need, but upon the health needs of her entire family.

Do You Really Need to Lose Weight?

Perhaps the desire to lose weight needs reevaluation. Statistically persons who are 20% or more overweight have more diabetes, heart disease, and many other health problems. For persons who are only five to ten pounds overweight, the purpose for losing weight may be primarily cosmetic. Be serious about answering this question: "Is God interested in my losing weight or am I merely listening to the voice of my cultural value system?" It may be better not to be concerned about that extra five or ten pounds because once on the dieting merry-go-round it is very difficult to get off, and a worse weight problem may be the unhappy result. Sue tells how she made this mistake while pregnant with her first child. She was so worried about gaining more than the allotted 20 pounds that she began to count calories and plunged herself into years of merry-go-round counting and yo-yo weight fluctuations. Only the Eating Better Lifestyle, high in dietary fiber and low in fat, rescued her and stabilized her weight.

What About Compulsive Eating?

The Eating Better Lifestyle does not cure compulsive eating behavior. It may assist to curb behavior that has a physiological basis such as an addiction to sugar, but behavior rooted in emotional needs may require special counseling. There are several Christian ministries from which you can get additional support. The restraint of sensual indulgences (Colossians 2:23) can only come by way of an inner work of the Holy Spirit.

Am I a Victim of "Fat Genes"?

Some despairing hearts cry, "All I have to do is look at food and I gain weight!" Why is that? The answer may partly lie in the "fat gene" theory. It may be possible to inherit a physical tendency to produce more, rather than less, fat cells. The clue to such a condition is fat relatives. Yet many cannot lay claim to a fat family. They also battle with weight because the refined American Diet has contributed to a fat-producing metabolism. Metabolism determines how the body burns calories. Aerobic exercise can alter body metabolism. Exercise contributes to both weight control and total health. It is nutrition's twin.

For further reading we recommend *Beyond Diet* by Martin Katahn, Ph.D. Katahn's two basic rules for weight control are in harmony with the Eating Better Lifestyle: 1) Avoid low-calorie diets; and 2) Adopt a high-fiber, low-fat diet.

IF YOU'RE SICK 'N TIRED OF BEING FAT

If you're sick 'n tired of being fat,
a whole foods diet is where it's at!
Low fat and high fiber, too—
You have everything to gain but weight,
in view.

High fiber calories pass on through
while many a fat one becomes part of you!
Whole foods chewing takes longer in time;
you'll find their calories more
satisfying.

While refined carbohydrates are a pasty
mess
creating addictions that do not
bless,
Succulent fruits and vegetables many
add vitamins, minerals, and pure water
plenty.
These you need to regulate
all the processes of body
to properly use what you ate.

More nutrients will more energy devise
and you'll feel more like exercise.
You'll do more work, and get more done.
Your metabolism will pick up and begin
to run.

Give yourself time—this is a slower way,
but it will last for many a long day.
God looks on the heart,
not on external appearance.
Thus seek total inner health with
prayer and perseverance.

27

Exercise: Nutrition's Twin

Do you not know that in a race all the runners
run, but only one gets the prize? Run in such a way
as to get the prize.

1 Corinthians 9:24

Gone are the days of necessary walking, climbing, running, and sweating to do our daily work! In twentieth-century America we have a unique situation in the history of
mankind that conspires against healthy bodies at normal
weights—a high-fat, low-fiber diet inadequate in vitamins
and minerals plus sedentary lifestyles. Yet our best hope for
utilizing most effectively the good food we eat for the total
health needs of our bodies is aerobic exercise. Since our work
does not provide it, we must create it for ourselves. In general, Christians have recognized and understood the value of
exercise for health much better than the nutritional value of
whole foods. The result is that we have ample exercise resources available to us through Christian ministries. Therefore, we will address this need only briefly.

What is aerobic exercise? Simply, it is exercise that increases the oxygen supply in the body and increases the rate
of body metabolism. This is valuable to health in many ways.
Benefits, most of them interrelated, may include:

Improved blood cholesterol level
Normalized blood pressure
Stabilizing of emotions—lowered depression,
    anxiety, tension
Increased physical energy and vitality
Increased alertness
Improved elimination

Detoxification through removal of toxic wastes from
body cells
Healthier cardiovascular system—heart, lungs, etc.
Improved utilization of food nutrients
More effective weight loss and maintenance control
of weight

Find the type of aerobic exercise that best suits your own circumstances and interests. There are plenty of ways to do it. Check church and community resources for group activity. For exercise at home there are excellent music and video tapes available. We have listed some below. Exercise with a friend who lives nearby. It is a great way to maintain mutual accountability and enjoy a conversation break in a busy day.

Emilie walks at least two miles a day, six days a week. She uses the time to pray. Sometimes she sings and just enjoys the beauty around her. The time passes very quickly and she's doing two things at one time. Occasionally she will invite a friend to walk with her just to enjoy each other's fellowship. It takes her 30 minutes to walk two miles. The benefits are great. Good exercise gets her heart rate up, gives her a sense of well-being, and releases stress.

Brisk walking is usually the easiest and most available exercise for everyone, and it is safer for women than jogging. A brisk walk is between 3½ and 4 miles per hour. Buy an inexpensive stopwatch to time your distance. Walking costs no money and provides a sunshine treat at the same time. In city areas many indoor shopping malls have distances marked off for walkers and provide the safety of on-duty security. On rainy days use a cassette exercise tape indoors for variety. *Beyond Diet* explains thoroughly how aerobic exercise will alter body metabolism.

If you are overweight, adopting the Eating Better Lifestyle will probably not help you to lose weight on a permanent basis without a regular discipline of aerobic exercise. Make three 20-minute sessions of aerobic exercise your minimum goal each week on alternating days. Incidentally, aerobics is not just for the overweight person. Everyone needs it!

Resources:

The Alternative Workout, video cassette (VHS or Beta) with Carolyn Cilley, Alternative Workouts, Inc., P.O. Box 33308, Phoenix, Arizona 85067.

The Better Better Body Book, Marge Frank and Nancy Linton, Zondervan, 1985—purchase at or order through Christian bookstores.

Exercise albums and videotape by Marge and Nancy—descriptions and order blanks at back of *The Better Better Body Book*.

Exercise For Life, Stormie Omartian, aerobics on record or cassette tape to music with or without exercise instructions during tape. Available at local Christian bookstores.

28

Drink Your Way to Health

Everyone who drinks this water will be thirsty
again, but whoever drinks the water I give him will
never thirst. Indeed, the water I give him will become a spring of water welling up to eternal life.

John 4:13,14

America's Unquenchable Thirst

America loves to drink everything but water—soda pop,
fruit drinks, fruit juices, alcoholic beverages, coffee, and tea.
We guzzle 50 million cans of Coke and 200 million cups of
coffee daily. How can plain water possibly compete?

Water Works!

Approximately three quarts of water are lost from the human
body daily through the kidneys, lungs, and skin. It must be
replaced continually to effectively perform the work of nutrient transport and elimination of wastes. Two-thirds water
by weight, the body thirsts for nontoxic, clean water, an
increasingly scarce commodity. Agricultural and industrial
wastes have polluted many public water sources. Chlorine,
added to kill bacteria, is a health hazard itself. Sodium fluoride, added to protect our teeth from decay, may also be
detrimental to health.

What Kind of Water is Best?

Fresh fruits and vegetables supply part of our water re-
quirement. The water in fresh produce is the purest kind. We
can heartily thank our Lord for it. Where, however, is our best
source of drinking water?

First, find out the quality of your tap water. Locate a water laboratory that will give you a chemical analysis. Check the yellow pages under "Laboratories-Analytical." An EPA-certified lab has been inspected by EPA and checked for testing accuracy. If the report lists any of the following chemicals, especially at toxic levels, you should consider an alternative drinking water source: chlorine, sodium fluoride, nitrites, arsenic, barium, cadmium, lead, silver, cyanide, coliform bacteria, or selenium. What alternative sources are best?

Alternatives to tap water include bottled spring water, distilled water, filters on faucets, reverse osmosis, and so on. The options are many and varied. It is often difficult to assess which is most economical, safest, and most effective. We are most familiar with distilled and bottled spring water. Some nutritionists suggest that distilled water leaches minerals from the body over a prolonged period of time. Others insist that it does not and that distilled water is our only guarantee of pure drinking water. We are not satisfied with either view. On the other hand, death rates are statistically lower in hard water areas. The lower death rate is attributed to the higher mineral content in hard water. Yet there can be harmful substances in the hard water, as well. We have chosen to use distilled water, adding mineral seawater purchased from the health food store. This provides us with a pure water source and the minerals we may possibly need. We add one to two tablespoons mineral seawater to five gallons of distilled water, an amount that will not affect the taste. If you purchase distilled water, purchase steam distilled and not distilled by deionization. Your tap water may also be distilled with one of the many home distillers.

If you choose spring water, it is wise to have a chemical analysis of it just as you would your tap water. If you have a water softening system in your home, using it for cooking and drinking is unwise.

The cost of any pure water source is more economical than the American Diet drinking budget!

Should You Drink Water with Meals?

Many health-food enthusiasts tell us not to drink water with meals because it dilutes the digestive juices in the stomach needed to digest food properly. Yet telling most Americans not to drink anything with meals is like telling a man dying of thirst in the hot desert to leave his water flask unopened! So let's be realistic about it. If you want something to drink with the meal, water is to be preferred over soda pop, fruit drinks and juices, and coffee. Keep the risk of diluting digestive juices in mind, however. Sip it a little at a time instead of gulping it or sloshing down food with it. You will discover quickly that the Eating Better Lifestyle that includes lots of fresh fruits and vegetables will not create as much thirst as meals high in meats and salt. Try drinking water without ice cubes. The body seems to prefer temperatures that are not extreme. Enjoy a refreshing slice of lemon in it. Lemon will help to purify the water.

How Much Should You Drink Between Meals?

Few people drink more water than they need. Usually we must tell ourselves that we need it. If you are a non-water drinker, drink one more glass of water a day than you now drink for a week. Increase it by an additional glass per day each week until you are up to 4 - 8 glasses per day. If you do not care for the taste of your water, it may be the combination of chemicals and minerals in the tap water. Many people purchase bottled water just for a better taste. A good idea if it encourages you to drink more!

I Must Have My Morning Cup of Coffee!

That morning cup just gives me the get-up-and-go, the energy, the alertness, and the vigor to start my day! Do I have to give it up?

Nutritionally, coffee has nothing to offer. It stirs up the nervous system, but does not build strength. Research suggests a mixture of blessings and curses from coffee drinking.

Reactions appear to be highly individual. Most troubles begin after the third cup, or about 200 milligrams of caffeine consumed within a 24-hour period. The following reactions are good reasons for quitting or cutting back on the caffeine habit: heartburn or gastrointestinal discomfort, irregular or increased heartbeat, high blood pressure, insomnia, irritability, a need to increase the amount in order to experience a sense of well-being, withdrawal symptoms such as headache and excessive fatigue or depression, frequency of urination, and diarrhea. Those who have ulcers, fibrocystic breast disease, high blood cholesterol, or are pregnant would be wise not to drink it. Coffee also consumes thiamine (B_1), and iron which can aggravate an anemic condition.

Some of coffee's effects are related to ingredients other than caffeine. For example, the oil caffeol can irritate the stomach lining, and chlorgenic acid can burn up some of the body's thiamine and iron stores. Decaffeinated coffee also contains these ingredients. Therefore, it may not be the best coffee replacement. Although some people worry about the chemical used to decaffeinate coffee, it generally does not get into the coffee. An alternative, however, is Swiss or water-processed coffee (available at health food stores if not the supermarket).

The caffeine habit can be broken gradually or cold turkey. Expect withdrawal symptoms with the cold-turkey method. These probably won't last more than a day or two. Start diluting each cup with a little water, increasing it to half a cup. Lowfat or nonfat milk added to coffee will weaken its acidy abrasiveness in the stomach. Cremora or Coffee-mate contain sugar and are not good substitutes for real milk. Reduce or omit sugar or substitute half as much granulated fructose. Gradually move on to black tea and finally to herb teas. A short fast up to three days can often break the craving for caffeine.

Take Time for Tea

Although black tea also contains caffeine, it has some advantages. Black tea can help alleviate mild headache, depression, and fatigue without as many risks as coffee. For example, black tea has not been found to raise blood cholesterol. Some of the properties in black tea can actually be beneficial according to "A Drink The Day After," *American Health Magazine*, April 1984: Polyphenols in tea work with vitamin C to strengthen blood vessel walls. Tea can inhibit growth of decay-causing bacteria in dental plaque, helps to fight colds, helps to minimize effects of radiation, and contains zinc, manganese, and potassium. It can reduce iron absorption, however. This is not a license to drink ten cups a day! But it is an improvement over coffee. Tea contains $1\frac{1}{2}$ to 2 grains of caffeine per cup as compared with 2 to 4 grains in a cup of coffee depending on how strong each is brewed.

Herb teas are safe and enjoyable in moderation. Each herb contains different medicinal properties. Some of them, if consumed to excess, can cause reactions. It is best not to drink many cups of the same kind. Teas made from peppermint, spearmint, and rose hips are good. The many supermarket blends are fine in moderation (2 or 3 cups a day). Peppermint can sooth mild stomach discomfort, and chamomile can be very soothing for mild headaches.

To make teas, pour boiling water over a tea bag or 1 teaspoon loose tea and let it steep for 5 minutes. Remove the tea bag or loose tea before you drink it. Iced herb tea can be delightful, too. To make sun tea put 2 tea bags per quart of water in a covered glass jar and set it outdoors in the sun for a few hours.

Juice It!

"We've quit the Kool-Aid, but we still get confused between juice drinks and juice. What's the difference?" Juice drinks are a blend of water, sugar, and perhaps 10% real juice. Fruit juices are all real juice, either unsweetened or sweetened. These all keep company on the same shelf in the supermarket. Read labels carefully to select the real and unsweetened juices. Bottled juices are to be preferred over canned. Unsweetened frozen juice concentrates, also occupying cozy quarters with the sweetened variety, are also good choices.

Even real juices are refined foods because they have been extracted from the whole fruits. This removes the dietary fiber and concentrates the sugar, even if it is natural. That doesn't mean to quit drinking real fruit juice. It is an improvement over soda pop and fruit drinks, but juice can't match the value of fresh fruit. Dilute fruit juice 50-50 with water to cut the sugar concentration and halve the price!

Fresh fruit and vegetable juices are in a class by themselves. None of the enzymes or other nutrient values have been destroyed by canning. Although the dietary fiber, along with a bit of the nutrients are removed, fresh juices can be very beneficial in cleansing the system during a short fast of up to three days. Dilute them also with water.

29

Mind, Mood, and Food

Love the LORD your God with all your heart and
with all your soul and with all your mind.

Matthew 22:37

Does Food Affect Mind and Mood?

"After Thanksgiving dinner I felt like taking a l-o-n-g winter's nap!" We can say amen to that! The effects of nutrients on the brain is a fascinating new field of research and experimentation. Judith J. Wurtman, Ph.D. has published an entire book on the subject, *Managing Your Mind And Mood Through Food* (Rawson Associates, New York, 1986). Nutrients do indeed affect mental clarity, emotions, and behavior. For example, starchy carbohydrates eaten alone will stimulate the release of serotonin, a neurotransmitter in the brain. Serotonin produces calmness and sleepiness. In contrast, protein suppresses the serotonin and wakes you up! Nonstarchy carbohydrates such as leafy greens, broccoli, and brightly colored fresh fruits don't affect the level of serotonin either way. Wurtman suggests that you eat protein with starchy carbohydrates to stay awake and alert. Eating food low in fat and not overeating is also important for a clear mind. That means save the spaghetti for dinner to relax afterwards and eat the tuna and lettuce on rye for lunch for a more mentally alert afternoon. Wurtman explains that this is the general pattern, but there are individual exceptions.

Does Food Affect Criminal Behavior?

Alexander Schauss, director of the American Institute for Biosocial Research and author of *Diet, Crime, and Delinquency*, has been instrumental in changing the nutritional quality of foods offered to prison inmates. The rates of recidivism (return to crime) have dropped significantly among juvenile delinquents and criminals who have been given better food. Says Bernard Fensterwald, III, NNFA Legislative Counsel: ". . . massive consumption of refined carbohydrates and other questionable substances by prison inmates causes severe behavior problems. Undeniably, they are more aggressive—which leads to more assaults, homosexual rapes and the like. At a minimum, they are continually disoriented and often act irrationally. Their ability to concentrate is impaired, and this lessens the prison's rehabilitation effort."[1]

Nutritional Therapy?

Research into the therapeutic use of food nutrients is demonstrating their value to health far beyond what we have traditionally understood. Nutrients in a variety of research projects have helped persons who are mentally retarded, mentally ill, emotionally disturbed, autistic, senile, juvenile delinquent, criminal, and slow learners. Almost all of the nutrients have been used in megadoses in varying ways and combinations, most notably the B-vitamins. Orthomolecular research is a branch entirely devoted to the nutritional approach to mental problems.

Does Nutrition Keep a Mind Healthy?

The effect of nutrition on mental behavior is currently viewed with skepticism by conservative scientists and researchers. For example, the value of the Feingold diet and the value of reducing refined sugar to fight hyperactivity in children have both been recently challenged. Yet the early evidence that nutrients are vital to mental health and behavior is promising.

We have introduced this aspect of nutrition to further inspire you to develop the Eating Better Lifestyle. If persons with such mental afflictions as we have mentioned are being helped by nutritional therapy, we wonder how many of these afflictions could be minimized or prevented by the Eating Better Lifestyle. It is becoming clearer that our minds and emotions depend upon physiological and chemical reactions in our bodies. "Love the Lord your God with all your . . . mind" (Matthew 22:37) suggests that doing those things which enhance our potential to respond to God's Word and to the indwelling Holy Spirit are worthy of our attention.

30

But I Love My Chocolate!

"Everything is permissible for me"—but not everything is beneficial. "Everything is permissible for
me"—but I will not be mastered by anything.

1 Corinthians 6:12

The hardest things to give up are those that we love! We can find all sorts of rationalizations for hanging on to them. Will it help a little if we say that you can "have your chocolate cake and eat it, too"? That's right! The white flour and the white sugar may be worse than the chocolate in it. You can make chocolate cake with whole wheat flour and honey. In fact, in home baking you can use chocolate in any recipe along with other ingredients that are more nutritious. But if you want to buy commercial sweets with chocolate you are in trouble! Chocolate keeps company with nutritionally unsavory ingre-dients! So if you love chocolate candies and other commercial chocolate creations, we suggest that you set a goal to prepare more wholesome homemade goodies even if they do contain chocolate.

In spite of your chocolate love we want to introduce the benefits of carob. Carob does not aggravate skin problems, contribute to digestive troubles, or cause allergic reactions as chocolate frequently does. Chocolate is especially high on the list of allergens, while practically no one reacts to carob.

Carob belongs to the legume family of beans and peas such as lentils and split peas. Therefore, it shares similar nutri-tional benefits. Carob is an excellent source of calcium, potas-sium, pectin and bowel-regulating dietary fiber, and contains iron, vitamin A, and vitamins B_1 and B_3. It does not contain the oxalic acid of chocolate that could interfere with calcium absorption and is not high in the stimulant theobromine.

Unlike chocolate, it is virtually fat and caffeine free. Carob has some of its own natural sweetness while chocolate is bitter. Therefore carob requires a little less additional sweetening in recipes.

Note how 3 tablespoons of carob powder compare with their equivalent of 1 oz. of chocolate:

	1 oz. Chocolate*	3 Tbsp. Carob
Calories	185	47
Fat	15.8 gr. (142.0 calories)	0.33 gr. (3.0 calories)
Calcium	20 mg.	90 mg.
Theobromine	1,047 mg.	0.4 mg.

*Hershey's Baking Chocolate

Chocolate is not totally devoid of nutrients. It does contain vitamin A, B-vitamins, and also more iron and potassium than carob.

What about the flavor of carob? We won't pretend that carob tastes just like chocolate. It doesn't—especially not to chocolate lovers! Rich, Sue's husband, as a chocolate lover, was not interested in the flavor of carob during the first year of transition to the Eating Better Lifestyle. Sue's daughter, Sharon, still does not care for carob. Yet her home-baked creations that include chocolate also include whole wheat flour, honey and other ingredients nutritionally superior to commercial goodies. A halfway measure is a blend of half carob and half chocolate.

Carob is easy to substitute in any recipe. Mix 2 tablespoons hot water with 3 tablespoons carob powder to replace each 1 oz. square of unsweetened chocolate. If cocoa powder is added to the dry ingredients, substitute the same amount of added to the dry ingredients, substitute the same amount of carob powder. Buy roasted carob powder in either the supermarket or the health food store.

In your favorite chocolate cake recipe substitute whole wheat pastry flour for half or more of the white flour. Use half as much honey as sugar. If you are not satisfied with the results, it may be better to start with new recipes already adapted to more nutritious ingredients (see page 287 for information).

31

Alterations for Allergies

There is . . . a time to search and a time to give
up, a time to keep and a time to throw away. . . .
Ecclesiastes 3:1,6

Do You Really Have a Food Allergy?

The symptoms of allergies or food sensitivities are often
confused with symptoms of other health conditions. Many
authorities believe that the number of Americans suffering
from true allergies is rare. Yet many do seem to get relief from
such problems as tiredness, lack of energy, mental confusion,
depression, crying spells, headaches, irritability, nasal drip,
mucous in the system, rashes, hives, and a host of others by
detecting certain offending foods in the diet. Any of the
following, however, could be causing allergy symptoms: the
American Diet; lack of exercise, rest, sunshine, fresh air,
plenty of drinking water, or peace with God through Christ;*
an unhappy relationship; unresolved emotional problems; a
serious disease; the need for vitamin-mineral supplementa-
tion; wrong food combinations; or allergies to nonfood items
in the environment. Therefore, the detective work to rule
out food allergy or sensitivity could easily be a misdirected
search. This fact is worth keeping in mind.

How to Find a Food Allergy

A health care professional may suggest some type of allergy
test. These can be expensive and are not always accurate.

---

*See *Greater Health God's Way* by Stormie Omartian

There are less expensive, do-it-yourself methods such as utilizing the elimination diet (*Tracking Down Hidden Food Allergy*, William G. Crook, M.D.) or the pulse test (*The Pulse Test*, Easy Allergy Detection, Arthur F. Cocoa, M.D.). There are others, as well (see Recommended Reading list, p. 284).

Common food allergens are milk, wheat, eggs, corn, potatoes, tomatoes, citrus fruits, carrots, chicken, beef, peanuts, apples, oats, green beans, soy, and yeast. The first four are the leading allergens in America. Often a problem food is one to which you are addicted.

Coping with a Food Allergy

After you have omitted a problem food for a month or more, start adding it back into your diet. Do not reintroduce more than one food at a time. Wait four days in between. If previous symptoms return, omit the food again. If some of the foods do not cause the old problems, you may be able to add them back into your diet. It is best not to eat them more frequently than every four days, however, if you do not want them to become problem foods again.

A fast of up to three days with at least two quarts of pure water or fresh fruit or vegetable juices a day, can be helpful. Sometimes certain food combinations can be too stressful on sensitive digestive systems. Try eating your fruits alone. Eat protein only with nonstarchy vegetables. Eat the starches such as cereals, breads, grains, and beans with nonstarchy vegetables only.

Keep in mind, especially if you are sensitive to many foods, that your condition is not necessarily irreversible. Some foods you may never be able to include. Others you can begin to enjoy with care.

Ingredient Alternatives

The four leading allergens are used in many different recipes. Our recipes in the *Eating Better Cookbooks* (see p. 287 for information) include ingredient substitutions for persons sensitive to milk, wheat, corn, and eggs. For wheat there are several tasty wheatless recipes using other whole grains. Use apple or pineapple juice in place of milk in almost any baking recipe. For milk-based soups you can use vegetable, beef, or chicken stock—add potatoes for thickness. Use the blender to make creamy nonmilk soups. You may be able to tolerate yogurt better than milk. If you are lactose intolerant, a digestive aid may help (p. 94).

Corn allergy need not be an obstacle in home cooking. Low-sodium baking powder does not contain corn and you can use arrowroot powder in place of cornstarch. These last two items are available in health food stores. Yeast can also have corn in it, but Red Star brand does not. If you are allergic to yeast, use quick bread recipes such as whole grain muffins, cornbread, and popovers. Sourdough and sprouted breads digest more easily and you might be able to handle these better. Some persons allergic to wheat can tolerate wheat in the sprouted form.

While wheat is a leading allergen, gluten intolerance—a rather severe reaction to gluten in grains—is not so common, but possible. The best cookbook reference we have seen for gluten-free cooking is *Good Food, Gluten Free* by Hilda Cherry Hills, Keats Publishing, Inc., New Canaan, Connecticut, 1976.

For egg alternatives see p. 88.

32

Ode to Pesky Preservatives and Poisonous Pesticides

Spray the crops to grow more than we need;
  refine them before the people we feed.
    Dress them up with color and taste;
    of good whole food, what a waste!

  How much preservative I can't tell.
    But it is added to everything
      so that it might sell.
  If you want food, pesticide free,
    you can grow your own
      for a very small fee.

    Some places you can buy it
        organ-i-cal-ly.
      Speak to the farmer,
      speak to the grocer,
  speak to the health food store owner.
    You'll find a supply, by and by,
      if you are but willing to try.
    Watch at the supermarket—
      some might be sold there.

Organically grown food is going to increase
        year after year
    because of what farmers now know—
      pesticides and fertilizers do their
        bank accounts wear low!

    So you and I can persevere.
    We may get better food one year.
    Organic foods may cost a bit more
    when we buy them from the store;
    but of purer food we'll not be poor.

142

And whatever those thousands of additives be,
of them all we can be free.
Just read those labels
and buy food that is whole
and be healthier
in spirit, body, and soul!

Organically Grown

Organic food is generally defined as grown without the use of pesticides and commercial fertilizers. There are various certification programs that set standards for certification of products. If food is labeled organic, request certification documentation. Insufficient legal documentation does not mean that it is not organic. It means you must trust the integrity of the farmer, wholesaler, and retailer.

33

Questions Often Asked

A man finds joy in giving an apt reply—and how good is a timely word!

Proverbs 15:23

Are you nutritionists?

No. Our focus is on homemaking. We do this by teaching principles of healthful living and how to apply them in the home to kitchen and household organization, shopping, menu planning, and food preparation. As such we are the women of Titus 2:3-5 who ". . . train the younger women to love their husbands and children, to be self-controlled and pure, to be busy at home, to be kind . . ."

The title of nutritionist usually designates a person who assists others who have specific health problems to set up individualized diet programs. Nutritionists frequently use various kinds of tests to determine an individual's dietary needs. They often work with a medical doctor, especially one who focuses on preventive care. The doctor will provide the diagnosis and the nutritionist then provides the diet program. Our menus and recipes serve as resources for the nutritionist.

Do you have a diet for diabetics?

Many people want a therapeutic diet for a disease or health condition. The Eating Better Lifestyle is adaptable to therapeutic diets. For example, our recipes call for honey, but a diet for a diabetic will limit the amount used depending on one's specific need, or suggest a special kind of honey, such as Tupelo honey. Therapeutic diets are designed with the help of a health professional such as a preventive care medical doctor or nutrition consultant. A worthwhile reference for the home library is *How To Get Well*, by Paavo Airola. Airola gives brief and clear dietary considerations in alphabetical order for 56 common degenerative diseases and health conditions.

Is fasting safe and should I do it? Is it a good way to lose weight?

Fasting is safe if done properly and has many benefits. It can be valuable in gaining control over a weight problem, but we do not recommend it as a primary means for losing weight. See "Why Diets Don't Work," (p. 119) and "Prayer and Fasting" (p. 171). Anorexia is an extreme form of fasting to prevent weight gain.

Are herb teas a good substitute for caffeinated beverages such as coffee, black tea, or cola drinks?

Yes. (See p. 130.)

If I quit using iodized table salt, will I get enough iodine?

This question belies the source of most Americans' nutritional education—advertising. Few are worried, for example, about getting enough magnesium. We worry about iodine, however, because the label on the iodized salt box states that "iodine is an essential nutrient." Table salt was iodized originally to compensate for iodine deficiency of the soil in the Great Lakes region. The soil is not iodine deficient everywhere. Seafoods, both plant and animal, contain iodine. Kelp is one of the richest sources and some people choose to use it in place of salt in cooking. It is an excellent choice. If you do not care for the taste, it can be added to the diet in tablet form. Sea salt that has not been kiln dried does not contain the RDA of iodine, although it contains traces. Seawater that might be added to distilled water (p. 128) contains iodine. We have chosen not to use iodized table salt; but if you want to use it for security, we do not consider table salt a health risk when used according to the Eating Better Lifestyle guidelines we have suggested (p. 115).

What do you think of NutraSweet?

We suggest caution in its use. (See p. 110.)

What do you think about microwave ovens? Do you have recipes for the microwave?

Sue has unanswered questions about the safety of microwave ovens. She has no adequate data, however, to advise against their use. Emilie owns a microwave and loves it. The general understanding is that microwaving preserves nutrients, especially in vegetables. We suggest two safety measures: 1) Do not stand in front of the oven while food is being cooked; 2) Have your oven tested periodically for leakage.

Generally, owners of microwave ovens do not take advantage of their full potential. A microwave oven can be a wonderful asset to whole foods cooking and especially for the working person. Recipes can be prepared in advance, or the evening before serving, and warmed quickly in the microwave after work. It just takes a little forethought, but virtually no additional preparation time.

Our recipes do not give microwave instructions. Microwave ovens differ. Follow the basic principles of adaption given in a good microwave cookbook or the book that accompanied your microwave oven.

I have heard that honey has more calories than sugar and causes tooth decay. Is this true?

Honey has slightly more calories than sugar. One tablespoon of honey has 64 calories compared to one tablespoon of sugar's 50 calories, but such a comparison is not practically meaningful since honey is twice as sweet. One-and-a-half teaspoons of honey will sweeten as well as one tablespoon of sugar, so in reality you consume fewer calories.

As for tooth decay, it would be more accurate to say, "Excess honey can cause tooth decay." When we teach about the value of using honey in place of white refined sugar, we are not suggesting excessive use of it. We do not suggest that a person substitute an average intake of 125 pounds of sugar, for example, with 125 pounds of honey, or even 63 pounds of honey. We suggest using it in quite small amounts. We ought to brush our teeth and teach our children to brush their teeth shortly after eating anything containing sugar, other than fresh fruits.

What do you think of food combining?

Those who advocate food-combining rules (p. 41) try to give what they believe is a scientific basis for it. But we are not fully satisfied with the explanation. Ruth Bircher in *Eating Your Way To Health* presents the position of the Bircher-Benner Clinic in Zurich, Switzerland: "We have tried to study this problem in detail but neither have we found sufficient facts which could be considered scientifically conclusive, nor have we found in our own clinical experience sufficient reasons for giving such general rules for the feeding of healthy people or invalids. Therefore, we do not feel justified in renouncing in principle all those natural, time-honored and valuable tasty combinations of healthy foods, such as 'potatoes and cream cheese', 'milk and cereals', 'apples and bread', which are all forbidden by these schools of thought. Such combinations are found particularly in the diets of the healthiest people in food geography or history . . . The incompatibility of certain foods is, in our opinion, something which has to be considered very carefully with each individual invalid by examining his reactions in each particular case. But it is really concerned with the invalid diet of the individual patient, not with the general teaching of dietetics."[1]

There are persons, however, who have been helped by adopting a diet based on food-combining guidelines. They have experienced more energy, better digestion, and help with weight loss and control. It is worthy of individual consideration, but we do not advocate it as a general pattern essential to the Eating Better Lifestyle. Many of our recipes are properly food combined or adaptable to proper food combining for those who want to follow that pattern. Limited food combining is a very difficult pattern for most Americans to adopt. Such loved dishes as spaghetti and meat balls, cheese pizza, hamburgers, lasagna, cereal with fruit, eggs, and toast, and pancakes with syrup are not allowed on such a diet. The all-American cheese or tuna sandwich is out of the question even if you do use whole wheat bread and cheddar cheese or water-pack unsalted tuna with dark green leafy lettuce and sprouts! We believe it is an unrealistic approach for most Americans. " 'People's food habits change very slowly,' say most anthropologists."[2] We believe the challenges that we have presented for change are more important for most people than food combining.

Should I drink water with meals?

With some caution. (See p. 129.)

Isn't margarine healthier to eat than butter? I thought butter was saturated fat.

Butter is saturated fat, but margarine is not a better choice. (See p. 77.)

What do you think of salt substitutes?

We don't believe salt substitutes are necessary. Usually the flavor of salt substitutes leaves something to be desired. (See p. 115.)

I just love ice cream. Is there anything healthier I can eat that can take its place?

Yes, there are some good frozen yogurts. Ask shops that sell frozen yogurt to show you the ingredients label of their product. Try to avoid refined sugar and a long list of chemicals. Make sure the yogurt is prepared with live bacteria culture (p. 94). We prefer that honey and/or fructose be used in it. If the nutrient data is listed, you can figure out the fat content. This isn't so important if you only eat it on occasion, but if it is a regular dietary item, a check on the fat content would be wise. Below is an example of how to figure the amount of fat:

1 gram fat = 9 calories.
4 oz. (½ cup) frozen yogurt = 4 grams fat
Therefore, 9 x 4 = 36 calories of fat.

4 oz. frozen yogurt = 140 calories
Therefore, 36 ÷ 140 = .26 or 26%
The fat content of the yogurt is 26% of the calories.

If the fat content is 30% or less in calories, it is within the Eating Better Lifestyle recommended range.

I've heard that it is not a good idea to use a lot of oil because it is so high in fat. What about olive oil?

Olive oil is an excellent choice (p. 78). Balance it with the use of some polyunsaturated oil such as sunflower or safflower oil. Olive oil is low in linoleic acid, an essential fatty acid. Polyunsaturated oils are a good source of linoleic acid.

I am hearing about "irradiated" foods. What are they? Are they safe to buy?

Food irradiation is becoming an important issue. Irradiated food is food treated by radiation to disinfect it, increasing shelf life from days to weeks. It may also destroy insects such as the Mediterranean fruit fly, reduce the need of spraying foods with chemical preservatives after harvesting, reduce the need for nitrates and nitrites in foods, destroy trichinosis organisms in pork, curb salmonella in poultry, and reduce botulism in cured meats. The FDA accepts the relative safety of irradiation and its advantages over whatever low risks there might be.

Irradiated food is not radioactive. But according to *Nutrition Action Healthletter*, "It cannot be stated with certainty that irradiated food is dangerous—or safe."[3] There are several reasons for this uncertainty. Various animal tests show conflicting results. More complete studies are needed. Some nutrient loss may occur at higher doses of irradiation than the FDA is now considering.

Mass irradiation of our food supply may be delayed by the controversy. Foods being considered for irradiation include wheat, fish, poultry, pork, beef, fresh fruits, and fresh vegetables. The current irradiation labeling law permits irradiated foods to be sold without careful labeling. At present, irradiated ingredients can be used in packaged foods and in restaurants without labeling. Labeling should be made clear on all food products so consumers can make informed choices. For more information about the food irradiation issue, contact: Health and Energy Institute, 236 Massachusetts Avenue, N.E., Suite 506, Washington, D.C. 20002, (202) 543-1070; or National Coalition to Stop Food Irradiation, Box 59-0488, San Francisco, CA, 94159, (415) 56N-CSFI.

Is aluminum cookware safe? I have heard that aluminum causes Alzheimer's disease.

Highly acidic foods such as apples, tomatoes, or recipes with apple cider vinegar, lemon juice, or other citrus juices are best prepared in non-aluminum cookware and stored in something besides aluminum foil. Other foods, however, probably do not absorb any significant amount of aluminum. Aluminum used in food products is of greater concern since the concentration is many times higher than what might come from aluminum pots. Our choice of cookware is stainless steel waterless cookware.

Alzheimer's disease has been related to high aluminum levels in some studies, but no conclusions have been reached.

Most diseases are the result of a combination of causes.

What is the best food for babies?

The best food for a baby is a well-nourished mother and father before conception. If you have not yet begun a family, adopting the Eating Better Lifestyle for yourself and your spouse is the best foundation. When the baby is born, mother's milk is superb. A well-nourished baby on mother's milk should not need any solid food before six months of age. Solids may be introduced between six and 12 months, but mother's milk is still the main food.

Introduce only one food at a time and watch for any negative reactions before adding a new food. Do not force-feed any food a baby rejects. Baby's digestive system is sensitive and allergies can develop easily. Start grains only after one year. By six months of age table food ground in a baby food grinder or blender provides better food than jars of commercial baby food.

For more information about feeding babies or small children, write to Eating Better with Sue (p. 287). See also p. 112, "Honey for Babies?"

Can you suggest a good magazine that will keep me abreast of the latest nutrition information?

Yes. *The Nutrition Action Healthletter*, Center for Science in the Public Interest (CSPI), 1501 16th St., N.W., Washington, D.C. 20036, (202) 332-9110.

What do you think of frozen vegetables? Are they good to eat?

Choose fresh vegetables as much as you can, filling in with frozen vegetables for variety. Frozen vegetables are much to be preferred over canned vegetables where nutrient loss is greater.

How do home-canned fruits and vegetables fit into the Eating Better Lifestyle? I have a large garden.

By all means preserve excess garden produce! There is a proverb: "Go to the ant, you sluggard; consider its ways and be wise! It has no commander, no overseer or ruler, yet it stores its provisions in summer and gathers its food at harvest" (Proverbs 6:6-8). Fruits can be canned in a honey syrup instead of using white sugar. Use half as much honey as you would sugar in a light syrup. Jams can be made with mild-flavored honey or granulated fructose. Recipes for strawberry or apricot preserves, peach or apple butter are available in *Eating Better Lunches & Snacks* (See p. 287 for information).

Choose freezing fresh produce over canning. You might also want to consider a dehydrator as an alternative to canning. Dehydrated fruits and vegetables preserve more nutrients than either freezing or canning.

34

The Value of the Human Body

> When I consider your heavens, the work of your
> fingers, the moon and the stars, which you have set
> in place, what is man that you are mindful of him,
> the son of man that you care for him? You made him
> a little lower than the heavenly beings and crowned
> him with glory and honor.
>
> Psalm 8:3-5

Of all God's creative works one is very special—man and woman created in His image. The psalmist sang, "For you created my inmost being; you knit me together in my mother's womb. I praise you because I am fearfully and wonderfully made" (Psalm 139:13,14). The human being is awesomely complex.*

Yet twentieth-century Christians elevate the value of the spirit over the body almost universally. The body is finite. The spirit is eternal. The result is that Christians consider bodily care less important than spiritual care. John White describes our misunderstanding in *The Masks of Melancholy*: ". . . most of us possess a muddled mixture of Greek and Hebrew thought which we have inherited in part through Plato, Aristotle, the Gnostics, St. Thomas Aquinas and the philosopher Descartes. We have divided the human being up into a less important physical part (body and brain) and a more important immaterial part (mind and soul)."[1] White's illustration of the interdependence of body and spirit is illuminating: "To compare mind with body is like comparing

---

*For an appreciation of the human body read *Fearfully and Wonderfully Made* and *In His Image* by Dr. Paul Brand and Phillip Yancey.

153

music with the pianist's fingers. 'What matters is the music!' we cry. Of course. But no fingers, no music. Clumsy fingers, bad music. Weak fingers, feeble music."[2]

Scripture teaches that when one receives Christ, the Holy Spirit comes to dwell in his/her body. The human spirit does not leave the body to dwell with God. Instead, the Holy Spirit comes to live in the physical body of the new believer (1 Corinthians 6:19).

Another mistake we have made is to view the human body as somehow evil. The apostle Paul said, "I know that nothing good lives in me, that is, in my sinful nature" (Romans 7:18). The King James Version of the Bible uses the word "flesh" instead of "sinful nature." We have misunderstood "flesh" to mean the physical body—"No good thing dwells in my physical body." This is entirely incorrect! Man's sin nature is the condition of his spirit, not his physical body! The body is subject to sickness, decay, and death not because it is sinful or evil in itself, but because it is a victim of man's sinful nature.

The body, on the other hand, is God's key instrument through which He communicates Himself to the world. It should be self-evident, therefore, that He wills for us to take care of our bodies wisely, conscientiously, and faithfully. It should be no surprise that God has put into nature a complex nutritional fueling system for this purpose.

A wise owner of a new automobile will heed the instructions of the operations and maintenance manual, written by the auto manufacturer to insure its optimum performance. The car owner will not select the wrong fuel in order to save time, money, or effort. God has also given us an instruction manual for our incredible human body machines. The first instruction is to understand ourselves as whole persons, not as disembodied spirits. New Age philosophy would like to separate bodies from spirits, but God does not. Even the separation of our bodies from our spirits at death is temporary. On resurrection day, the dead in Christ will be raised to life—new bodies reunited with their spirits. Those alive in Christ will have their decaying living bodies changed to imperishable ones. We will all sit down (in physically new bodies just like Christ's resurrection body in Luke 24:40-43) at the wedding banquet table with the Lamb of God—our Redeemer, Jesus Christ—and dine on food!

Throughout this book we have already made application of God's Word to the subject of food. In the following chapters we want to add a bit more from God's "Instruction Manual." We cannot exhaust the subject, but want to raise awareness so it will be clear that our foundation for the Eating Better Lifestyle is solid biblically. While this may not appear important on the surface, it is vital because we are surrounded by approaches to diet and health that oppose the purpose of the Christian life.

35

God Has a Plan for Health

He forgives all my sins and heals all my diseases;
he redeems my life from the pit and crowns me with
love and compassion. He satisfies my desires with
good things, so that my youth is renewed like the
eagle's.

Psalm 103:3-5

The Bible is our most important health manual. Our God is truly our Great Physician. The Old Testament health laws, the restoration of Job to health, the healing ministries of the prophets Elijah and Elisha, our Lord's own healing ministry, and the promise of an eternity without sin and sickness all attest to God's plan for healthful living. "There can be no question that Jesus Christ regarded illness as something to overcome. He did not acquiesce to it. He did not ignore it. He did not content himself with making the best use of it, important as this is when illness is not removed. He coped with illness, and he conquered it. It was his teaching that God wills healing, and he interpreted his healing acts as signs of God's power in the world and of God's ultimate intention to redeem the whole man."[1] When the leper came to Jesus and said, "If you are willing, you can make me clean," Jesus replied, "I am willing . . . be clean" (Mark 1:40,41).

Creation is also a witness to God's powerful healing character. His ". . . invisible qualities—his eternal power and divine nature—have been clearly seen, being understood from what has been made, so that men are without excuse" (Romans 1:20). This means that even without the Bible man can see the power and holiness of God in nature. "Natural law is God's law, and the more we learn of physiological . . . processes the greater is our awareness of the vast intelligence of the Creator."[2] For example, He has put many mechanisms in our bodies both to protect us from, and to fight, danger and disease. Pain is a very useful physical response that not only keeps our fingers from getting burned on a hot stove, but insures that we will rest during sickness to give the body a better chance to heal. Pain signals that something is wrong so that we will seek a remedy. Sickness is our experience of the body's fight to stay well. Fever, for example, is caused by the war of the white blood cells against infectious bacteria. When a finger is cut or a knee is bruised, the body undertakes an intricate process of healing. Our bodies are designed to continuously operate for health and wellness. We also see that natural things such as food, water, and oxygen keep us alive. We know that the vitamin D from sunshine is needed for strong bones and teeth. Creation cries out with a loud message: "God is willing to heal sickness."

We cannot blame God then for sickness and death. The source of these lies elsewhere. Man subjected himself to sickness and death when Adam and Eve chose to rebel against God's command in the Garden of Eden. We have inherited a sinful nature. Because of our sinful nature we make wrong choices. Much personal suffering (though certainly not all) results from our own wrong choices. For example, the choice to smoke can result in lung cancer, the choice to drink excessively can lead to a diseased liver, the choice to eat refined food can lead to chronic constipation or to colon cancer. Much of our sickness and untimely death is inflicted by choices, including poor lifestyle choices. We are not merely ill-fated victims of such tragedies. Peoples of other cultures who eat native whole foods in their local environment do not suffer these tragedies. God has put standards for health into the creation and in His Word. He can expect Christians to heed them.

36

Prevention, Miracle, and Medicine

> . . . All healing is of God, whether it occurs through what we call natural law or according to laws which we do not yet know.[1]

For over one hundred years Christian medical missions have been operating throughout the world, but the people they serve are just as sick as ever. Medical missionaries are learning what many Americans are learning. Crisis medicine to cure illness does not remove the cause. Medical missions are now taking a close look at what is called Primary Health Care. Primary Health Care means establishing such things as clean water supplies, adequate food, nutrition, and sanitation. Primary Health Care is taking advantage of God's preventive measures for good health. It means following His health standards. That is what the Eating Better Lifestyle is all about. It does not provide the sensationalism of a miraculous cure. It means discipline and the challenge of planned work. Yet both of these means are equally from God. We should not ignore a healthy lifestyle until we get sick, and then go to the doctor to get "fixed up," or ask God for a miracle cure. God has given us the benefits of all three of these health means—prevention, miracle, and medicine. To carelessly ignore prevention and then cast our sick bodies at the feet of the doctor or at the foot of the cross for a miracle cure is no different than jumping off a building to see if God's holy angels will rescue us in midair (Matthew 4:6,7)!

Primary care for health begins in the home with proper nutrition, exercise, rest, meaningful work, love and acceptance, companionship, and moral standards. "The importance of home and family in the realm of physical and mental health is very great."[2] Making a plan and working a plan for eating better is essential to the complete Primary Health Care package.

37

Not Health for Health's Sake

> The Spirit of the Sovereign LORD is on me, because the LORD has anointed me to preach good news to the poor. He has sent me to bind up the brokenhearted, to proclaim freedom for the captives and release for the prisoners, to proclaim the year of the LORD's favor and the day of vengeance of our God.
>
> Isaiah 61:1,2

Why does our God want us to be in good health? Is it to make us happy, to make us feel good, to give us more time to do the things we want to do, to be spared the pain of sickness, to put off dying as long as possible?

Three examples will help us to put purpose for health into perspective. These three cases involve the lives of three persons deeply dedicated to promoting health through better nutrition: Nathan Pritikin, author of *The Pritikin Program for Diet and Exercise*; Adele Davis, forerunner of the current health food movement who wrote several books on nutrition such as *Let's Eat Right To Keep Fit*, and *Let's Cook It Right*; and Gladys Lindberg, founder of the Lindberg Nutrition Service and coauthor with her daughter Judy Lindberg McFarland of *Take Charge of Your Health*.

Nathan Pritikin

Nathan Pritikin, engineer by profession, educated himself thoroughly in nutrition and degenerative disease. He dedicated his life to helping persons find new health and longer life through his diet and exercise program, particularly persons with heart disease. He established the Longevity Center in Santa Barbara, California, and the Longevity Research Institute. Thousands of people have benefited from the Pritikin program. Senator George McGovern, at Pritikin's funeral, eulogized, "Nathan Pritikin was a man of great dedication, unusual humility, a bold pioneer, perhaps the greatest lifesaver that lived in the twentieth century."[1] Yet, when Pritikin learned that he had leukemia, he chose a drug treatment that further devastated his life. He committed suicide.

Adele Davis

Adele Davis' work in nutrition was ahead of most of the current health literature. For many years her books were the primary nutrition instruction for millions of people. Yet Ms. Davis died of bone cancer. She attributed the disease partly to her habit of smoking which she stopped two years before her death. Faced with sickness and death, Ms. Davis gave her life to Jesus Christ.

Gladys Lindberg

Gladys Lindberg has spent over 40 years of her life sharing the benefits of good nutrition to better the lives of millions of people. Adele Davis was one of her lifelong friends. Mrs. Lindberg writes in *Take Charge of Your Health*: "During her illness, I visited her frequently, and she, knowing my relationship with God, asked many penetrating questions. At last, she asked to be taken to a special religious service, and that day I saw this great lady surrender her life to Jesus Christ."[2]

For Nathan Pritikin, health was an end in itself. It was his life pursuit. When he learned that he no longer possessed it, he had nothing left for which to live. For Adele Davis, suffering from a degenerative disease was used of God to get her attention. She responded and recognized that physical health is not all there is to life. Gladys Lindberg ministered to more than Ms. Davis' physical need. Her loving friendship and faith in the Lord Jesus Christ opened the door for Ms. Davis. "Now this is eternal life: that they may know you, the only true God, and Jesus Christ, whom you have sent" (John 17:3).

God has given His children a mission in the world to reconcile people to the one true God through Jesus Christ. While Nathan Pritikin and Adele Davis ministered the benefits of God's natural law to others in the healthy years of their lives, neither was able to bring the life of God in Christ to people. The greatest glory of Ms. Davis' life was her recognition of Jesus Christ as her Lord and Savior. Yet, Gladys Lindberg's healthy life has been used of God to teach people not only how to use His whole food resources for better health, but also how to introduce them to the Lifegiver!

Why then should we concern ourselves with health? We are concerned so we can better minister the life that is in Christ to a hurting and hungry world. "For we are God's workmanship, created in Christ Jesus to do good works, which God prepared in advance for us to do" (Ephesians 2:10). Our God-given ministries and good works are many and varied. We need all the physical, mental, and emotional strength that food can supply to carry them out.

38

The Perfect Vegetarian Diet in the New Age

> Have nothing to do with godless myths and old wives' tales; rather, train yourself to be godly. For physical training is of some value, but godliness has value for all things, holding promise for both the present life and the life to come.
>
> 1 Timothy 4:7,8

There are sincere Christians who are enthusiastic advocates of vegetarianism and there are Christians who avoid it altogether because of its associations with Eastern cultic religious philosophy. There is a difference between a vegetarian diet practiced for nutritional reasons and cultic "vegetarianism." If we are vegetarian enthusiasts, we will want to avoid its cultic implications. And if we are skeptics, we will not shun the nutritional value of a potentially nutritious diet.

From the nutritional standpoint the vegetarian diet is quite sound and much to be preferred over the American Diet. We have already defined vegetarian diets (p. 40). We have introduced both problems of meat eating and of dairy products, and discussed the merits of the complex carbohydrates as our best foods in other chapters.

Cultic vegetarianism, on the other hand, is a religious practice that denies the Lordship of Jesus Christ, and it is antibiblical. For example the ". . . ultimate perfection of a vegetarian diet . . ." is ". . . eating only food offered to Kṛṣṇa . . ."[1] The cultic vegetarian who aims for this perfection will offer his food as a sacrifice to Kṛṣṇa before he eats it. Such food offered to Kṛṣṇa is called "*prasadam*, a Sanskrit word meaning 'mercy of the Lord.' "[2] We must not think that this "Lord" is our Lord Jesus! It is not! Christians can easily be misled by the concepts of cultic vegetarianism because not only is "the Lord" spoken of freely, but arguments from the Bible to prove vegetarianism are used. It is easy for us to be fooled if we are not discerning of the spirits. These arguments from Scripture are incomplete. For example, religious vegetarians will use them to "prove" that our Lord was a vegetarian, but they overlook such key incidents as Jesus feeding the 5,000 men with five loaves of barley bread and two fish (John 6:1-15), Jesus providing a large catch of fish for the disciples on two different occasions (Luke 5:4-6 and John 21:5,6), Jesus serving them fish for breakfast Himself (John 21:13), and eating fish Himself (Luke 24:40-43). In addition, the fact that Jesus fulfilled all the Old Testament law during His earthly life means that He inevitably partook of the lamb served yearly at every Jewish Passover feast.

Cultic vegetarians also twist the meaning of Genesis 9:4, "But you must not eat meat that has its lifeblood still in it," to mean that God commanded man not to eat meat at all. This is a direct contradiction of Genesis 9:3: "Everything that lives and moves will be food for you. Just as I gave you the green plants, I now give you everything." In addition, cultic vegetarians overlook the fact that God instituted the killing of animals as sacrifices for sin before the coming of Christ and that portions of the sacrificial meat and grain offerings were the dietary mainstay of the Levites who served God in performing the sacrifices (Leviticus 7:35,36). Certainly there were restrictions such as not eating the fat and the blood (Leviticus 3:17) and not eating several "unclean" animals forbidden for food (Leviticus 11), but even a weak case for nonmeat eating cannot be made from the Word of God!

Food that is acceptable to the cultic vegetarian must be sacrificed to Kṛṣṇa: "the material substance of food . . . becomes completely spiritualized."[3] Such spiritualized food, or *prasadam*, is helpful in achieving the goal of reawakening the soul's original relationship with God.[4] "The very simplest form of offering is to simply pray, 'My dear Lord Kṛṣṇa, please accept this food.' "[5] We can see that cultic vegetarianism is clearly a denial of Jesus' proclamation, "No one comes to the Father except through me" (John 14:6). The religious vegetarian preaches a false Christ.

The theology of religious vegetarianism does not correspond with scientific observation in the field of nutrition, either. For example, according to religious vegetarian theology, food is not classified according to carbohydrate, protein, fat, or its vitamin and mineral content—things that can be explained and observed by the rational mind. It is classified according to "goodness, passion, and ignorance."[6] "Milk products, sugar, vegetables, fruits, nuts, and grains are foods in the mode of goodness and may be offered to Kṛṣṇa."[7] Meat, fish, eggs, garlic, and onions are not acceptable to Kṛṣṇa.[8] Nor is food cooked "by people who are not devotees of Kṛṣṇa. According to the subtle laws of nature, the cook acts upon the food not only physically, but mentally as well. Food thus becomes an agency for subtle influences on our consciousness."[9]

We may think that this information is irrelevant to our interest in food, but we need to understand that while vegetarianism may have nutritional merit, the basis of its origin is not the Judeo-Christian tradition but Eastern Hinduistic religion that denies the gospel of Christ. Religious vegetarianism fits 1 Timothy 4:1-3 exactly: "The Spirit clearly says that in later times some will abandon the faith and follow deceiving spirits and things taught by demons. Such teachings come through hypocritical liars, whose consciences have been seared as with a hot iron. They forbid people to marry and order them to abstain from certain foods, which God created to be received with thanksgiving by those who believe and who know the truth."

39

The Great New Age
Health Deception

*The health food boom of the 60's that served up
bean sprouts and tofu salads along with exercise
has been infused with a sacred side.*

Carol McGraw
Los Angeles Times

In the last chapter we discussed religious vegetarianism, just one aspect of the New Age philosophy. New Age philosophy is based on the concept that God and man are one. Man has limitless potential that can be realized through tapping into all manner of supernatural sources. All is seen as good and useful to developing human potential. The purpose of developing human potential is self-realization.

What does this have to do with healthy eating? Much, in every way! Adopting a healthy diet can be approached in two different ways. One way is biblical. The other way is diabolical. This may seem like a strong term to use, but it is important to understand the difference.

The biblical foundation for the Eating Better Lifestyle is based on two truths: 1) The God of the Bible—Yaweh, Jehovah—the God of Abraham, Isaac, and Jacob is Creator and Sustainer of the Universe; and 2) The same God is the Redeemer through His Son, Jesus Christ. It is from Him, and Him alone that we draw our resources for life, both natural and supernatural. Our purpose is not to find self-realization but to obey Jesus Christ.

What has happened in the New Age Movement is this: People have begun looking for answers to ultimate health. One thing leads to another. Diet alone is not sufficient. More is needed. There is a whole world of supernatural benefits as well to tap into. For example, the theme of the Whole Life

165

Expo held in Pasadena, California, on February 6-8, 1987, was "Explore New Frontiers of Health and Self." The expo offered numerous seminars and workshops on how to utilize these supernatural avenues for health, along with the usual food and diet emphasis.

"They are becoming involved in a world of evil and ultimately in the whole realm of Satan's jurisdiction,"[1] says F. LaGard Smith, author of *Out on a Broken Limb*. An "almost common experience in American society"[2] today is delving into such realms as witchcraft, astrology, clairvoyance, mediumship, metaphysical counseling, trance channeling, astro-travel, crystals, and reincarnation. According to Andrew Greely, "four in ten Americans say they have had contact with the dead and 60% have experienced extrasensory perception."[3] The Christian rejects all supernatural avenues to health that God has forbidden in His Word. We have but one supernatural ave. ue, the Holy Spirit who lives in us.

Many diets assume a nonbiblical philosophy. We must be careful to distinguish between nutritional value and the religious trappings. For example, one of the coauthors of a well-researched and influential cookbook wrote:

> A mantram, very simply, is a name of the Lord, hallowed by the thousands of people who have repeated it. People have used some form of mantram in almost all the great religious traditions. 'Jesus, Jesus' is a mantram; 'Rama, Rama' is Gandhi's mantram. It seems paradoxical, but repeating the mantram has a way of keeping you planted firmly in the right here and right now, concentrated and calm. Not only that, but it helps you to remember all the while that you aren't just slapping together a meal; you're preparing food for the Lord in those you love.[4]

There is a proliferation of such antibiblical philosophy propagated throughout health food stores, cooking classes, television cooking shows, university extension classes, health magazines, health and nutrition books, cookbooks, and by health practitioners. We can easily be deceived because these resources 1) communicate much sound nutritional information; 2) use Christian terminology when speaking of "the Lord"; 3) work for the same apparent goals as Christianity such as peace and love; and 4) use the ploy that "It works." Christians have been especially drawn in by this latter philosophy, "It works." On the surface it appears innocent enough. But Christians must ask, "Is it based on what is biblically true?" It is easy to embark on a healthier lifestyle without understanding the basis for it. This is dangerous. There is more at stake than physical health. There is no way to have true or eternal peace and love, for example, except through faith in Jesus Christ. Every good work of our lives must be built upon that foundation—including the physical and practical matters such as diet.

40

Give Thanks

For everything God created is good, and nothing is to be rejected if it is received with thanksgiving, because it is consecrated by the word of God and prayer.

1 Timothy 4:4,5

"Bless this food to the nourishment of our bodies." Do we pray this prayer as a traditional hangover from Grandpa's generation or do we really mean it? Do we think that our prayer will somehow transform the nutritional value of the food? The word "consecrated" in the dictionary is defined as "set apart or dedicated to the service of the deity." When we give thanks for our food to God, our Creator and Redeemer, we acknowledge that He has created it and given it to us as a gift.

If we give thanks to God because He created the food for our nourishment, how important is it that it retain its nutrient value? If we give thanks to Him for giving it to us as a gift, is it right to turn the gift into something it wasn't meant to be? Let's be honest. We may be able to continue to give thanks to God for devitalized food in ignorance. But once we know what true nutritional food value is, can we honestly give thanks for inferior food when we know we could do better?

Let's be clear about one thing. Giving thanks for our food does not change its nutritional value, nor does it change the way our bodies will process it. Giving thanks from the heart to God is a health-giving action in itself, but it does not affect the physical nature of the food.

Everything God created is good. Our perversion of many of His good things is not cause for thanksgiving, but for repentance and change. Let us consecrate to His service food that reflects His creative purpose for it—our health and well-being for His honor and glory.

168

41

Dealing with Opposition

Let us not become weary in doing good, for at the proper time we will reap a harvest if we do not give up.

Galatians 6:9

"Are we going to have that weird stuff again, Mom?" "Here comes the health nut . . . I wonder what she brought this time!" "Is she trying to kill us?" "Gee, can't we go to McDonald's for dinner?"

You are convinced that the Eating Better Lifestyle is important for your family. You readily began the challenge with plenty of resources. You thought you were following all the "dos" of a winsome approach. Bam! The opposition comes. Are you ready for it? No matter how well and how carefully you pursue your plan, you will receive some negative responses. Your children may complain, your husband may be indifferent, friends may tease you, relatives may be offended, others may give you the cold shoulder. You know that what you are doing is right. You have done your research and made your commitment to God.

Why the opposition?

We travel a narrow road. The world food system consists of two approaches, both of them unbalanced—the hedonistic and the restrictive. The hedonistic approach to food is the American Diet sold to the public by big food corporations who don't care about your health unless it means more profit. Most of the profit is made by appealing to the lusts of the flesh, however. The restrictive approach challenges us with: "Don't use any salt. Don't use eggs. Don't use butter. Don't use honey. Don't eat fish. Don't use dairy products. Don't, don't, don't!" How can you weather the storms of criticism?

First, be fully convinced that developing the Eating Better Lifestyle is God's purpose for you based on the foundation of the Scriptures and on sound nutritional information. Second, find the support of another person. Third, bring each obstacle to God in prayer as it comes. Request His guidance for a workable solution and for His power to transform attitudes. Trust God to assist your efforts. Be on the alert for possible problems you may be causing yourself through a wrong approach or attitude. Sometimes God says "wait." If that happens, wait and "watch." Pray for the barriers to be broken and watch for the appropriate opportunities to begin anew. Do not give up because you meet opposition. It is the normal condition of a godly life.

42

Prayer and Fasting

> Is not this the kind of fasting I have chosen: to loose the chains of injustice and untie the cords of the yoke, to set the oppressed free and break every yoke?
>
> Isaiah 58:6

The Eating Better Lifestyle is not complete without the discipline of prayer and fasting. Most persons can safely fast once a week for 24 to 36 hours. Fasting gives the body an extended rest from digestion, helps to cleanse the body of toxic wastes, and serves to clear the cobwebs from the mind. A period of fasting can break a craving for a particular food, especially if the fast is of three days' duration or longer. A periodic fast of three days, three or four times a year, is safe for most.

Fasting provides a special opportunity for communion with God. It is a time to do spiritual battle to break through seemingly impossible barriers in your own or someone else's life.

To learn how to fast and how to prepare for problems that may arise during a fast, read at least one of the following:

Fast Your Way to Health by Harold J. Smith
God's Chosen Fast by Arthur Wallis
Greater Health God's Way by Stormie Omartian

43

Good Food Is Good for Love

> Better a meal of vegetables where there is love
> than a fattened calf with hatred.
>
> Proverbs 15:17

Mealtimes are the best times for family fellowship and communication. Children need family relationships expressed in the context of eating together. A survey was taken to discover what high school valedictorians had in common. One activity was found: Each ate one meal a day together with the family. Meals shared say "I love you" when Jesus Christ is the center of our relationships. They bind families together.

It is not easy for a family to enjoy quality meals together. The pervasive influences oppose it. The average American child views 8,000 to 13,000 food commercials on television per year—23 to 36 per day![1] The restaurant industry spent $930 million on advertising in 1984. Advertising has made deep inroads on the Christian family. We are so busy working to earn a living and doing work for the Lord in the name of Christian ministry, we have yielded the decisions about food value to the profit makers of our society. We have been sold a new value system based on taste, eye appeal, convenience, and nutritional half-truths. Approximately 42% of meals are now eaten away from home. The number of families who eat together even one meal a day is diminishing at an alarming rate.

What we have done in our churches with the Lord's Supper (Communion) is illustrative of our disregard for the central place that food can have in living the gospel of Jesus Christ. We now pass the wafer and the grape juice while our pastors illuminate their meaning from the Word of God. Yet our Lord instituted the Lord's Supper in the context of the Jewish

172

Passover meal. The first-century Christians celebrated it in the context of mealtimes. The essence of Jesus' death was not just expressed in a sermon, but experienced in the fellowship, communion, and intimacy of eating together. The "visible" food was an expression of the "invisible" nature of God. Romans 1:20 and Psalm 19:1-4 clearly express that God reveals His glory in physical realities. How then can we enhance the meaning of the gospel of Christ both in our own lives and to the world through our use of food? There are many wonderful ways!

Sharing the Gospel of Jesus Christ Through Food

Sharing healthful food is basic to a full expression of God's love. The unhealthy American Diet that leads to sickness and premature death is not in harmony with the life-giving gospel of Jesus Christ. "If Jesus truly nourishes us and the Lord's Supper is to remind us of that, we should eat food that truly nourishes."[2] The wife of Proverbs 31 was a business woman. She was a busy woman. Yet she did not neglect the affairs of her household. She brought her husband ". . . good, not harm, all the days of her life" (Proverbs 31:12). She brought her food from afar and provided food for her family (31:14,15). To do so today requires a careful selection of health-producing food for our spouses and our children, and also for every person with whom we share food. To offer any other kind of food is an incomplete expression of love.

"There is nothing that says lovin' like something from the oven," is one food commercial that speaks truth. Food can express love in a way that a thousand words cannot. Our Lord said, ". . . anyone who gives you a cup of water in my name because you belong to Christ will certainly not lose his reward" (Mark 9:41). He placed high value on physical provisions offered in His name. When food is shared in the name of Jesus Christ, it is not a mere excuse for evangelism. It is the gospel in action. There are many occasions for sharing food.

Every important celebration includes food: birthdays, weddings, funerals. Compassion and kindness can be extended

with food to the new neighbor, to a neighbor moving elsewhere, to a family with illness or the arrival of a new baby, to a
family experiencing a death, to a friend or neighbor who is
out of a job, or to the poor in the community. Churches enjoy
coffees, potlucks, fellowship meals, Sunday school refresh-
ments for children, women's luncheons, men's prayer breakfasts, and picnics. Some fellowships participate in organized
food ministries to the poor, to the sick, and to shut-ins.

These occasions do not require high-fat, low-fiber, devitalized food. Proverbs 15:17 explains why we do not need it:
"Better a meal of vegetables where there is love . . ." This
means that healthy eating is not merely a private affair. It is
not something to set aside on the way to the church potluck.
We do not need to reform the church by edict or by law about
food. But we can each begin to introduce whole foods to
believers through informal food-sharing opportunities. Moving the Eating Better Lifestyle out of our homes into public
ministry in our churches and among friends and neighbors
will not be easy. For many of us we will be alone in our
endeavors and often misunderstood, even teased or ridi-
culed—yes, even by fellow Christians! Yet such a commitment to the life-giving value of food is essential to the life-
giving ministries of the church. We need a "vision." Our
growing awareness and pioneer efforts in sharing whole
foods with others in all of these various situations can be
forerunners pointing to the ministry of the church worldwide
to people who are hungry, both physically and spiritually,
which we will discuss in the next chapter.

If you are a leader in your church fellowship—pastor, elder,
deacon, deaconess, women's ministries leader, hospitality
chairperson, head of a food outreach ministry, youth director
who plans youth outings and parties, a camp food manager,
ask God to give you a "vision" for bringing the life-giving
nutritional value of food to the ministry for which you are
responsible. Pastors, elders, and husbands who are not involved with food preparation need to understand the role of
food in the gospel of Jesus Christ and begin to support those
who are becoming nutritionally aware.

The mark of the church is the love of Jesus Christ expressed in ministries to hurting people. Peggy is a person "hurting" from a compulsive chocolate addiction. The church, on the one hand, offers ministries to persons like Peggy for coping with and conquering compulsive behavior. On the other hand, when Peggy finds chocolate brownies served at a church gathering she says, "It is like going to an Alcoholics Anonymous meeting and finding a bar there." We all love chocolate brownies, but we have disregarded the health needs of many brothers and sisters.

Food Sharing Opportunities

Jewish Feast Celebrations: Many Christians are reviving the celebration of Jewish feasts with a Christian interpretation— the Passover seder in the spring, the Feast of Tabernacles in the fall, and others. The Feast of Tabernacles can be celebrated in lieu of our American Thanksgiving (for information write Eating Better with Sue, p. 287). *Celebrate The Feasts* by Martha Zimmerman is an excellent resource. Eating Better Lifestyle recipes are easily adaptable to these celebrations.

Lord's Supper Celebration: Communion can be shared in the context of a meal with fellow church members in homes or in the church fellowship hall periodically. Whole wheat matzos could be served in place of communion bread or wafers made with white flour.

Potluck for the Poor: Share an inexpensive soup and muffin meal as a church fellowship periodically and take an offering for the poor or for a Christian organization that ministers to the needy such as World Vision or World Relief Commission.

Anniversary or Wedding: Serve a whole wheat wedding cake with cream cheese frosting. The decoration can be made with regular decorator icing. One of Sue's friends enjoyed a three-tiered wedding cake for 250 persons prepared from the Applesauce Cake in *Eating Better Desserts* (see p. 287 for information). Serve a trail mix, punch with real fruit juice, and vegetable relish tray with dip. Groom's cake can be whole wheat banana bread or fruitcake.

Birthday or Children's Parties: Serve whole wheat cake or cupcakes, real fruit juice punch, whole grain cookies, frozen yogurt, honey vanilla ice cream.

New Neighbor: Take a loaf of homemade whole wheat bread or muffins in a colorful basket.

Death in a Family: Skip desserts and take something basic so that those who are grieving do not need to cook, such as a hearty soup, muffins, a main dish salad, a casserole dish. Sue did not have to cook any meals for a full week following the death of her son, Stephen. Love shared in this way is a great blessing.

Unemployment: Share a "love basket" of something you prepare yourself or produce from the garden—a loaf of fresh bread, muffins, a pound of butter, a jar of honey, a batch of granola. Many do not appreciate handouts, so make it something fun and special rather than a basic bag of groceries until you discern the recipients' feelings. Then, if basic groceries are appreciated, make them better-quality items such as fertile eggs, water-pack tuna, Hollywood mayonnaise, peanut butter without hydrogenated fat and sugar, etc.

Home Schooling: The home school setting is a wonderful opportunity to learn about preparing and serving whole foods with children. Parents can learn at the same time.

Restaurant Meal: Take a small loaf of homebaked whole wheat bread to give to the waitress with a note of appreciation attached for her services.

Love Basket: All Christian marriages need rekindling with romantic moments. Fill a love basket for an overnight or a day's outing with favorite whole food recipes and foods.

Church Coffees, Potlucks, Classes, etc: Offer whole food alternatives. For example, serve herb teas alongside the coffee, real fruit juice in place of punch, fresh fruits or whole grain home-baked goods alongside commercial donuts and cookies.

If you take a tasty dish to a potluck such as a dozen Minute Bran Muffins, you'll influence 12 people with how tasty whole foods can really be. You will even get requests for recipes!

44

Christian Ministry
in a Hungry World

For he satisfies the thirsty and fills the hungry
with good things.

Psalm 107:9

The train lurched to a stop in the Mexican village. Young
girls rushed forward and eagerly held up to our window bags
of succulent mangoes. Imposing itself on the landscape behind
them loomed a Coca-Cola truck, the only vehicle in sight
parked on the single muddy village street. That one scene
captured the reality of what is happening worldwide. People
everywhere are being inundated by refined, devitalized food.

Wherever refined foods such as soda pop, white flour and
white sugar products, polished white rice, and canned foods
have traveled, the health of people has deteriorated. Cavities
and crooked teeth, diabetes, heart disease, cancer, and obesity
are the legacies of refined food. Research projects conducted
worldwide bear out the truth of this fact consistently.* Says
D. B. Jelliffe in *Nutritional Reviews*, September 1972, "The
food industry in developing countries has been a disaster . . . a minus influence."[1]

Why is this happening? It is happening because powerful
food industries are expanding their marketing of refined food
products throughout the world. People in other countries are
just as interested in convenience foods as are Americans.
Food from the West is also viewed as a status symbol. In
Africa, for example, many will shun the local whole grains in
favor of white rice.

---

*For more information, write Eating Better with Sue (p. 287).

The food industry not only influences the nutritional quality of food throughout the world, it also influences the economics and politics of supply. There is ample food to feed the world. Natural disasters and lack of land to grow food may appear to be the reasons for hunger, but they are not. The Institute of Food and Development Policy cites economics and politics as the root causes of hunger.

Why should Christians be concerned? The same influences that have created the devitalized condition of our food supply in America are traveling across the world. Many Christians travel throughout the world to take the gospel of Jesus Christ to other people. Most missionaries take the influences of the refined American Diet with them. In contrast, Charles and Edna Lewis, missionaries in Indonesia, have chosen to take full advantage of the local whole foods where they live. As a result, Charles can do the work of four Indonesian Christian men because he eats a nutritious diet. In addition, the Lewises have opportunity to share with their Indonesian friends the best use of the locally available whole foods. It is food for thought.

45

Planning Is a Privilege

Command those who are rich in this present
world not to be arrogant nor to put their hope in
wealth, which is so uncertain, but to put their hope
in God, who richly provides us with everything for
our enjoyment.

1 Timothy 6:17

The Israelites in the wilderness complained bitterly to
Moses: "If only we had died by the LORD's hand in Egypt!
There we sat around pots of meat and ate all the food we
wanted, but you have brought us out into this desert to starve
this entire assembly to death" (Exodus 16:3). How quickly
they forgot about their slavery in Egypt and the power of God
to deliver them. You may be wondering, too, as you develop
the Eating Better Lifestyle, "Is it worth it all?"

The Israelites were consigned to 40 years of eating manna
for their lack of faith in God's ability to provide for them.
Each day they were to collect what manna they needed—no
gardening, no harvesting, no storing of food, no grocery
shopping, no menu planning, no food preparation, no recipes to follow. Just the same thing to eat meal after meal—
"manna waffles, manna burgers . . . ba-manna bread . . ."![1]
If we lived in a developing country our food variety could be
limited and scarce. Which would we rather have—starvation
rations, only one or two foods to eat, or an abundance that
requires planning and discipline? Let us bless our God—not
with complaints, but with thankful hearts for the abundance
we must manage!

46

Meal Planning and Shopping

Make plans by seeking advice. . . .
Proverbs 20:18

Meal Planning Is Essential

Help! I've never been so bogged down and frustrated with meals, time, energy, and finances in my life. Everything has run away with me. I'm a mother of four children and one husband and I am a nurse attending a community college and active in our local church. But meals become a real headache. At 5:00 P.M. I fall apart. HELP! HELP!

We often receive a letter like this from busy moms. Meal planning can save headaches, stress, and even finances in homes. Emilie knows from the experience of feeding five children under five years of age, one husband, and many drop-in friends, family, and hungry people. Sue knows from feeding family, live-in students, and hundreds of campers. Mealtime can and will be a joy when, and only when, we plan ahead! It takes little time to save much time. HAVE A PLAN, WORK THE PLAN, AND THE PLAN WILL WORK FOR YOU.

How to Plan the Menu

Keep your menu plan simple by focusing only on the dinner meals for one week. First make a simple menu sheet: Fold an 8 ½ x 11 sheet of paper in half lengthwise. Fold it in half crosswise and in half again crosswise. You now have eight squares. Write the name of each day in each of the seven

181

squares.* Select a main dish for each square. Start with our 35-Day Unlimited Planned Menu or 20-Day No-Meat or No-Dairy Menus (pp. 223-25). Choose one to three new recipes. You can choose more, but don't overdo it. Space these new recipes between your regular familiar meals. After you have written in the main dishes you can add choices of vegetables, salads, and breads.

When you have finished the menu chart, decide on a few ingredient changes you can start making in your own favorite dishes. Choose from the list of Super Starter Steps (p. 190). Note these on the menu chart. For example, if you plan to use ground turkey in the spaghetti on Thursday evening, write "with ground turkey" in the menu chart square. If you are going to put darker leafy lettuce in the tossed salad on Monday evening, write "with dark leafy lettuce" under tossed salad in the square. If you are going to make any changes for breakfasts, lunches, or snacks, note them briefly in the eighth blank square on your menu chart. For example, you may note "new breakfast cereal," "raisins and sunflower seeds for snacks," "whole wheat bread for toast." Now you are ready to prepare the shopping list.

The Shopping List

Arrange your market list in the same order that food items are arranged in the market where you do most of your shopping. This will take you through the aisles of the market quickly. List all the ingredients needed for your main dishes. Most of the ingredients needed for our recipes can be purchased in the supermarket. Check the Shopping Guide (p. 196) for a complete list of ingredients used in the recipes in this book. A few of them that require a health food store are marked with an asterisk (*). Write the health food store ingredients on a separate list.

---

*Menu planning charts are also available in *More Hours in My Day, Survival For Busy Women,* and *The Eating Better Cookbooks* (See p. 287 for information).

Next, list the necessary fruits, vegetables, dairy products, breads, cereals, condiments, etc. needed for the balance of the dinner meals and for breakfasts and lunches. Include snack foods such as fresh fruits in season, dates, raw and unsalted nuts, carrots, zucchini (to cut into sticks), celery, cucumbers, turnip rounds. Include the new items listed in the eighth square of your menu chart.

Now work on your health food store list. You may be making your first trip to a health food store. Check "How to Locate Shopping Resources" (p. 218) if you need help in locating one. If you want to begin stocking your pantry with items from the health food store that are not on your menu plan, a beginner list is given on p. 198. In addition, you might want to take the Survey Check List (p. 199) with you.

Generally, health food stores are further from home. You can save extra trips later by shopping for staples in advance. But stick to our list of items on p. 198 unless you know exactly what you are going to do with other items you might purchase. Don't do like our friend Jamie, who gave away all her familiar pantry items and completely restocked the kitchen with health food store products she did not know what to do with. When they got bugs in them, she decided that she wasn't ready for that kind of cooking. She tried to do too much at once. Keep things simple. It is better to do one new thing well that will become a way of life than to do too many things and give up in frustration.

Include your family in preparing the menu and shopping lists. An older child can note down items to purchase as you plan menus with your husband and/or children. Children love eating what they have planned and prepared. This is part of helping the family to change. If you train them well, they can take over for you completely on frequent occasions when they get older (a super time-saving bonus!).

The Shopping Trip

Plan to shop the same day each week. Shopping will be more complex while starting the Eating Better Lifestyle. Once you have located your best resources, a pattern will develop. You will probably shop at more than one store—supermarket, health food store, dairy, local produce stand. You may need to make a second shopping trip during the week for fresh produce. Check the ads in your newspaper. Supermarkets restock periodically each week. Shop when produce items are available in fresh abundance. Eat beforehand so that you are not hungry. Keep to your market list and shop quickly. Women spend at least 75 cents a minute after the first half hour in the market, according to one study. Women who adhere to planned whole food menus and market lists save as much as $16-$20 weekly. If you are easily influenced by disruptive children or by their pleas for items not on your list, do not take them. Otherwise, use the time to teach them how to select fresh foods and packaged foods by reading labels (see p. 215). For example, if an item lists sugar as one of the first two or three ingredients, it is high in sugar. Find a similar item that has no sugar listed and show your child the difference. Suggest that together you buy fresh fruit such as bananas and raisins or dates for a no-sugar cereal. Gradually, your children will also understand that a few minor changes can turn the meals into better eating.

Further Help with Menu Planning and Marketing

Be consistent about the time you plan each week's menus just as you are consistent with shopping days. As you progress in developing the Eating Better Lifestyle, you will include more of our recipes and menus, and better ingredients in all your meals. We have given you several guidelines to menu planning and resources to help you in your shopping in Part 6. Use them.

47

Guidelines for
a Balanced Menu Plan

We would all like to know how we can plan menus to include all the nutrients that we need. Will we get enough calcium into our menus, enough protein, enough vitamin A, enough iron? The Recommended Dietary Allowances are put neatly into a chart to let the American public know how much of each accepted nutrient has been judged necessary by the National Research Council for normal health. Some nutrition books and cookbooks such as this one also include nutrient data—usually the total calories, fat, protein, and carbohydrates. In addition, we have included dietary fiber and calorie charts, as well as a list of best food sources for the vitamins and minerals. All of these can be of some help to give the idea of what we are looking for in our food. When it comes to actually planning the menu, however, we need simple and workable guidelines, focusing on the kinds and quantities of foods. We need to understand nutrition, but it is the food that we see, touch, smell, taste, and prepare. Here are three basic guidelines to assist your menu planning and shopping:

1. DAILY FOOD GUIDE (p. 186)
2. BASIC MENU PATTERNS (p. 188)
3. PLANNED MENUS (p. 223-25) (for dinners only)
   a. 35-Day Unlimited Menu
   b. 20-Day No-Meat Menu (Lacto-Vegetarian)
   c. 20-Day No-Dairy, No-Egg Menu

The *Food Guide* gives the general picture. The *Basic Menu Patterns* suggest the specific type of foods to use in meals. The *Planned Menus* give specific main-dish recipes.

FOOD GUIDE

Fresh Vegetables—think LOTS! think MORE, MORE!
    Especially dark leafy greens, cabbage, broccoli
    Especially dark yellow
    Some for lunch
    Some for dinner

Fresh Fruits—think TWO PIECES MINIMUM
    At least one citrus for vitamin C
    One for breakfast
    Best for snack or separate meal

Whole Grains, Beans and Peas—think MODERATE
    In combinations in main dishes or,
    Bean dish with bread, or
    Grain with milk or cheese
    Breads, cereals, muffins

Nuts and Seeds—think SMALL
    In baking, main dishes, garnishing
    Small snack

Dairy Products—think SMALL TO MODERATE
    Especially lowfat, nonfat, cultured

Eggs—think ONCE/TWICE A WEEK
    think IN BAKING OKAY

Meats and Poultry—think BITS 'N PIECES
    In casseroles, stir-fry, occasional "hunk"

Fish—think 1 TO 3 TIMES A WEEK (minimum)
    Especially fatty ones—salmon, mackerel, tuna

Fats—think TINY
    Butter on breads, oils for salads

Sweets—think SPECIAL OCCASION AND TREAT

How much to eat WHEN?

Breakfasts—think SUBSTANTIAL

Lunches—think SMALLER TO MODERATE

Dinners—think SMALLER TO MODERATE
think EARLY
think FAMILY TOGETHER

Snacks—think 1 OR 2
midmorning and/or midafternoon
fresh fruit, protein, vegetable munchie-crunchies

For Weight Control and Energy:

Spread your food out over the day,
fueling the body for work
and
not for hitting the hay.

BASIC MENU PATTERNS

BREAKFAST PATTERNS:

#1 whole grain cereal
    lowfat, nonfat milk
     or yogurt
    whole grain toast
    English muffin, or
     muffin
    fresh fruit piece

#2 egg
    whole grain toast
    English muffin,
     muffin, or
     coffee cake
    fresh fruit or juice

#3 pancakes/waffles
     or French toast
    fruit topping/
     maple syrup
    yogurt or milk

#4 fresh fruit salad or
     cut fruit wedges
    yogurt or cottage cheese
    crushed nuts, 1-3 tsp.

#5 protein shake
    whole grain toast
     or muffin (optional)

LUNCH PATTERNS:

#1 whole grain sand-
     wich or pita bread
    high protein or vegetable
     filling
    dark leafy lettuce
    veggie munchies
    milk or yogurt

#2 soup
    whole grain muffin
     or crackers
    veggie munchies
    yogurt, cottage
     cheese or cheddar
     cheese

#3 leafy green salad
    protein bits—egg,
     tuna, chicken, cheese,
     nuts, seeds, beans
    whole grain muffin
    milk (optional)

#4 fresh fruit salad or
     cut fruit wedges
    yogurt or cottage
     cheese
    crushed nuts, 1-3 tsp.

LUNCH PATTERNS: cont.

#5 protein shake
whole grain muffin

DINNER PATTERNS:

#1 main dish, meatless
green or carrot salad
fresh vegetable, cooked

#2 main dish with/meat
green or carrot salad
fresh vegetable, cooked

#3 fish, chicken, turkey
brown rice dish
green salad
fresh vegetable, cooked

#4 main dish, cheese
green salad
fresh vegetable, cooked

#5 soup
whole grain muffin
hot bread/crackers
veggie munchies

#6 fresh fruit salad
yogurt or cottage cheese
crushed nuts, 1-3 tsp.
whole grain muffin
(optional)

#7 protein shake
whole grain muffin
or bread

#8 egg dish
green salad
fresh vegetable, cooked
whole grain muffin,
toast, or English
muffin

#9 large fresh salad
high-protein filling
hot whole grain bread
or muffin

ACCOMPANIMENTS: Up to 1 Tbsp. butter with breads/day, 1½ tsp. honey or unsweetened jam occasionally, 1½ tsp. to 1 Tbsp. oil salad dressing or up to ¼ cup yogurt or buttermilk-type dressing

48

Super Starter Steps
to Improved Meals

Here's how to make nutritional improvements in your own favorite meals beginning in your own supermarket and with simple food preparation changes.

—Begin to replace at least half the iceberg lettuce in tossed salads with darker leafy lettuce such as romaine, green leaf lettuce, or ruby red lettuce. Include at least four other fresh vegetables in tossed salads.

—Replace processed cheeses such as American cheese with cheddar, jack, or mozzarella cheese. Try to reduce the amount called for by 1/3.

—Replace regular cottage cheese with lowfat cottage cheese.

—Use ground turkey in place of ground beef in all your favorite burger dishes. Season it before browning (see recipe, p. 234).

—Use turkey breakfast sausage (Louis Rich brand, for example) in place of pork sausage or bacon for breakfast.

—In salads and sandwich spreads, replace half the mayonnaise with nonfat or lowfat plain yogurt. Buy mayonnaise that is made without chemical additives or sugar (Hollywood brand, for example).

—In recipes calling for sour cream, replace half or all of it with nonfat or lowfat plain yogurt, or use Lite Sour Cream (Knudsen Nice 'n Light).

—Use peanut butter made without hydrogenated fat and sugar.

—If a recipe calls for cream cheese, use Neufchatel cheese instead. It is lower in fat.

—Use brown rice in place of white rice. If not ready for this, choose Uncle Ben's Converted Rice in preference to other white rice. More nutrients are retained in processing converted rice. Try mixing half white rice and half brown rice.

—Purchase bulgur wheat (also called Ala) to use in any meal in place of rice. Bulgur is parboiled wheat that cooks in a few minutes or may be soaked instead of cooked. Follow package directions.

—Use half or more whole wheat flour in baking.

—Purchase only whole grain cold cereals without sugar added such as Shredded Wheat, Grapenuts, NutriGrain cereal.

—Purchase only whole grain hot cereals such as Quaker Oats, Wheatena, Zoom, Roman Meal.

—Cut fat in recipes in half, replacing shortening with oil or butter, or with half oil, half butter.

—Purchase at least one fresh vegetable from the cabbage family each week to include in the menu such as cabbage, broccoli, brussels sprouts, kohlrabi, or cauliflower. There is something that is in these vegetables that helps to protect against cancer—maybe beta carotene or maybe some other yet unidentified nutrient or combination of them.

—Replace distilled vinegar with apple cider vinegar.

—Use Kikkoman Milder Soy Sauce to season in place of regular soy sauce or salt in casseroles, soups, and main dishes where it blends well. One tablespoon milder soy sauce contains 510 mg. sodium as compared to 942 in regular soy sauce and 2,131 mg. sodium in one teaspoon salt.

—Buy carrots with the tops still attached. Place tops with ends of spinach, broccoli, parsley, and other vegetable scraps saved in a Ziploc bag for a week or less in a large pot. Barely cover with water, boil 3 minutes, reduce heat and simmer 2 hours. Strain and refrigerate or freeze the broth for use in soups.

—Purchase salad dressings with real food ingredients and no sugar or chemical additives, such as Newman's Own Olive Oil and Vinegar Dressing.

—For beef dishes such as stroganoff calling for cubes or strips, use flank steak. It is the lowest fat beef cut. Ask butcher to tenderize it for you. Marinate in one tablespoon Kikkoman Milder Soy Sauce blended with one tablespoon arrowroot or cornstarch for several hours.

—When buying tortilla chips, look for those made with stoneground cornmeal and vegetable oil that is not hydrogenated. Some supermarkets will carry them.

—Cut sugar in recipes in half, replacing it with honey. Reduce oven temperature by 25°.

—Saute vegetables in a little water instead of fat.

—Cut salt called for in recipes by 1/3 and see how they taste.

—Use lowfat or nonfat milk instead of whole milk.

—Substitute buttermilk or nonfat yogurt thinned

to buttermilk consistency in place of sweet milk in baking.

—Add fresh veggies to tuna or egg salad sandwich filling such as chopped celery, onion, green pepper, cucumber, grated carrot.

—Prepare mashed potatoes, potato salad, and fried potatoes without removing skins.

—Add a few canned kidney and/or garbanzo beans to tossed salad for added protein, fiber, vitamins, and minerals. Canned beans are high in sodium, but are convenient to use in small amounts. Rinse them well before adding.

—Remove skin from chicken and turkey.

—Trim all visible fat from meats and poultry before cooking.

—If making a meat, chicken, or turkey broth, refrigerate to let the fat rise to the top. Skim off fat before using.

—Buy unsweetened real fruit juices for breakfasts, snacking, and sack lunches (juices without sugar or high fructose corn syrup or sweetener).

—Use fresh garlic and fresh onions liberally. Buy a garlic press. One garlic clove replaces ¼ teaspoon garlic powder.

—Use garlic powder and onion powder in place of garlic salt and onion salt.

—Cut amount of meat called for in a casserole by ⅓. Increase the amount of vegetables by ⅓.

—Purchase at least one bunch of dark leafy greens to include in the menu each week such as kale, collards, spinach, chard, mustard greens.

49

How to Improve
a Popular American Meal

The menu is:
Lasagna
Tossed Salad
Garlic Buttered French Bread

The American version of lasagna contains ground beef, cottage cheese, cheese, and lasagna noodles made with white flour. The tossed salad consists of mostly iceberg lettuce with a garnish of red cabbage and tomato wedge topped with Thousand Island dressing. The bread is white bread with margarine.

What can be done to this menu to transform it into an Eating Better Lifestyle menu? First, the lasagna. Omit the ground beef, or cut the amount in half and use very lean ground beef, or better, use ground turkey. Omitting the meat altogether would be the best. Instead of American cheese and regular cottage cheese use cheddar or mozzarella cheese, reducing it by one third, with lowfat cottage cheese. Use whole wheat lasagna noodles, or omit noodles and use zucchini slices. Add a little onion, some green pepper, a little carrot, and maybe a head of steamed and chopped spinach.

Now for the salad. Use at least half darker leafy lettuce such as romaine and green leaf, and ruby red. Add at least four or five vegetables not used in the lasagna. For example, add chopped celery, radishes, cucumber, alfalfa sprouts, and jicama. Serve it with olive oil and vinegar dressing.

In place of the bread or lasagna noodles serve lightly cooked broccoli or frozen green peas. If the noodles were omitted from the lasagna serve a whole wheat French bread or bake delicious Minute Bran Muffins. Both lasagna noodles and bread are not needed in the same meal. Use real butter with the bread.

Eat more of the salad and enjoy the cooked vegetable. Eat less lasagna which is higher in fat than the bread because of the cheese in it. Whole wheat lasagna noodles are much more filling than white flour noodles anyway. The whole grain bread is more filling, too, so eat less of that if it is served.

The meal will be more attractive because it has more color variety. It will have more variety in texture and contain more vitamins and minerals. In place of refined carbohydrate it will contain a substantial amount of dietary fiber and be lower in fat. There will be more to chew so that the family will stay at the table to enjoy one another's company longer. Finally it will be less expensive because the most expensive ingredients are omitted or reduced, and the lasagna will serve more people. By lowering the fat, reducing the amount of starchy carbohydrate, and not overeating we might leave the table to spend a quality evening with more alert minds!

Summary of the Eating Better Lifestyle menu:

Lasagna (with whole wheat noodles)	Lasagna (with zucchini)
Dark Leafy Green Salad	Dark Leafy Green Salad
Cooked Broccoli or Peas	Cooked Broccoli or Peas
	Minute Bran Muffins

You can take simple measures like this to transform many typical familiar meals. Soon you will have many Eating Better meals!

50

Shopping Guide for Recipes

The following items are used in the recipes in this book. Items that are normally only available at health food stores are marked with an asterisk (*). Fresh foods (fruits, vegetables, dairy products, tofu, meat, fish, poultry) are not included. All fresh food ingredients can be purchased at the supermarket.

Grains, Flours, Pastas, Cereals:
____brown rice
____pearled barley
____rolled oats
____unprocessed bran (wheat)
____whole wheat flour
____*whole wheat grain noodles
____*whole wheat spaghetti
____*stoneground cornmeal

Dry Beans:
____ lentils
____ black-eyed peas
____ kidney beans

Nuts:
____almonds (raw, unsalted)
____cashews (raw, unsalted)
____walnuts

Dried Fruits:
____raisins
____dates or *date dices (not sugar coated)

Frozen Vegetables:
____Corn
____Peas

Canned Food Items:
____diced chilies
____sliced ripe olives
____water chestnuts
____stewed tomatoes
____tomato sauce or tomato pieces
____dry minced onion
____mushroom stems and pieces
____garbanzo beans

Canned Food Items: cont.

_____unsweetened pineapple juice

_____unsweetened pineapple chunks

_____unsweetened crushed pineapple

_____water-packed tuna

Cooking Supplies:

_____soy sauce (Kikkoman milder)

_____apple cider vinegar

_____olive oil

_____lemon juice

_____mayonnaise (Hollywood)

_____salsa

_____garlic cloves

_____unflavored gelatin

_____baking soda

_____vanilla extract

_____cornstarch or *arrow-root powder

_____honey or *unheated, unfiltered honey

_____*ketchup (without sugar)

_____*chicken broth

_____*low sodium or Rum-ford baking powder

Cooking Supplies: cont.

_____*carob chips (unsweetened)

_____*granulated fructose

Herbs and Spices:

_____bay leaves

_____Italian seasoning

_____chili powder

_____cinnamon

_____cumin powder

_____cayenne pepper

_____garlic powder

_____ginger

_____marjoram

_____nutmeg

_____onion powder

_____oregano

_____paprika

_____rosemary

_____sage

_____sweet basil leaves

_____thyme

_____tumeric

_____*sea salt

_____*Instead of Salt Fish Seasoning (Health Valley)

_____**Bernard Jensen's Natural Vegetable Seasoning

**Bernard Jensen's Natural Vegetable Seasoning - not essential but given as a delicious variation in some recipes; made from soy, wheat, alfalfa, corn; low sodium; a yellow powder; often hard to find, but worth it if you can find it. See p. 218 for mail order source.

51

The Health Food Store

You will find many additional food items in health food stores that are not available or are more expensive in supermarkets. Begin to investigate the resources. Take the Survey Checklist (p. 199) with you. Supermarkets are most deficient in whole grain flours, pastas, and breads. The following items are a basic beginner list to stock your pantry:

—whole grain bread
—whole wheat spaghetti, lasagna noodles
—low-sodium baking powder
—sea salt (see p. 115 and p. 218 to mail order)
—cold pressed or unrefined safflower or sunflower oil
—granulated fructose (1 lb.)
—chicken and/or beef broth
—alfalfa seeds (for sprouts—see p. 113)
—whole wheat pastry flour
—stoneground cornmeal
—Spike seasoning (great seasoning—half salt, half other herbs and spices)

SURVEY CHECKLIST FOR THE
HEALTH FOOD STORE

(Make several copies of this list. Visit more than one store. You'll soon know what is available and where to shop.)

Whole Grains: ___wheat ___pastry wheat
___rolled oats ___oat groats ___millet
___buckwheat ___triticale ___rye
___amaranth ___short-grain brown rice ___corn
___long-grain brown rice ___basmati rice ___wild rice
___quick brown rice ___quinoa ___barley

Whole Grain Flours: ___winter wheat (bread flour)
___pastry flour ___oat flour ___millet flour
___buckwheat flour ___triticale flour ___amaranth flour
___cornmeal ___brown rice flour ___wheat bran
___oat bran

Whole Grain Cereals: (list 4 you would like to try)

_____

_____

Whole Grain Pastas: ___spaghetti ___macaroni
___noodles ___lasagna

Whole Grain Crackers and Chips: ___whole wheat
___rye ___brown rice cakes ___grahams
___stoneground corn chips ___blue corn chips

Whole Grain Breads: ___sandwich bread ___pita breads
___English muffins ___hot dog buns
___hamburger buns ___dinner rolls ___French rolls
___whole wheat tortillas
___stoneground corn tortillas or chapatis

Whole Grain Mixes: ___ cake___muffin ___nut bread
___pancake ___cookie

Beans: ___ soybeans ___ lima beans ___ kidney beans
___black (turtle) beans ___pinto beans
___garbanzo beans ___ black-eyed peas___mung beans
___azuki beans ___split peas ___lentils
___red beans ___navy beans ___great northern beans

Nuts: ___almonds ___pecans ___cashews ___walnuts
___peanuts

Seeds: ___sesame seeds ___sunflower seeds
___alfalfa seeds ___poppy seeds ___flax seeds

Spreads: ___peanut butter (salt only)
___peanut butter (no salt) ___almond butter
___tahini (sesame) spread
___jam (honey or unsweetened) ___pure maple syrup

Baking Items: ___low-sodium baking powder
___sea salt ___nonfat dry milk powder
___carob powder ___unsweetened coconut
___roasted carob powder ___arrowroot ___carob chips
___unrefined oil
___cold pressed oil ___blackstrap molasses
___honey (unheated, unfiltered) ___honey
___granulated fructose ___date sugar
___liquid lecithin (to grease pans)

Condiments and Cooking: ___apple cider vinegar
___soy sauce ___mayonnaise ___ketchup
___pickle relish (honey sweetened or unsweetened)
___salsa ___mustard ___salad dressings
___salad dressing mixes
___Bragg Liquid Aminos (like soy sauce, but milder in
flavor and lower in sodium)

Dried Fruits: ___raisins ___date dices ___apricots
___apples ___pineapple

Beverages: ___herb teas ___coffee substitutes
___natural sodas ___mineral water

___Swiss process decaffeinated coffee
___bottled juices (unsweetened)
___fresh vegetable juices (refrigerator)

Canned Goods: ___spaghetti or pasta sauce
___chicken broth ___beef broth ___soups
___chili con carne ___vegetarian chili

Spices and Seasonings: ___Spike
___Fish Herb Seasoning (Health Valley)
___Bernard Jensen's Natural Vegetable Seasoning (yellow powder) Other:_____

Meats, Poultry (organic or without chemicals): ___beef
___chicken ___turkey ___ground turkey

Packaged Meats (without nitrates, nitrites, or sugar):
___chicken weiners ___turkey weiners
___luncheon meat

Dairy: ___nonfat yogurt ___lowfat yogurt
___buttermilk ___goat's milk ___kefir
___raw certified milk ___raw certified whipping cream
___tofu ___kefir cheese ___low-sodium cheddar cheese
___raw certified cheese ___goat cheese
___raw certified butter ___honey ice cream
___frozen yogurt ___fertile eggs
___tofu sandwich spread

Frozen Foods (of interest to you): ___vegetables ___fish
___prepared entrées

Fresh Produce: ___organically grown? ___large selection
___small selection

Food Supplements: ___wall-to-wall? ___bee pollen
___brewer's yeast ___psyllium seed

52

Dining Out

How can I continue my Eating Better Lifestyle when I eat out? The first step is to develop this mentality: "I am in control." You do not need to be a victim of food fare in public places! Sometimes the whole food offerings are few, but with a little forethought and discipline you can plan your strategy. How does one evaluate food quality? The answer to that question is to define the Eating Better Lifestyle and look for those characteristics in public eating places.

High Fiber

Salad bars with a wide variety of fresh vegetables; some include fruits as well; look for the dark leafy greens among the iceberg lettuce. The FDA has banned sulfites to preserve freshness of salad ingredients, but ask about it anyway. Public places do not always adhere to new rulings right away.

Make the salad bar your main dish. Additions of sunflower seeds, alfalfa sprouts, cottage cheese (lowfat, when possible), grated Parmesan cheese and kidney and garbanzo beans can be added for protein.

Main dish salads such as chef's, tuna, chicken, vegetarian, or taco. You can request ingredients to be left out or exchanged. For example, ham can be omitted from a chef's salad. Water-packed tuna can be used in the tuna salad. Chicken is often an option in a taco salad, and you can ask for less meat in it and more of the garden ingredients with a reduced supply of the chips.

Fresh Fruit-In-Season Salads plain or with plain yogurt or lowfat cottage cheese or a bit of cheddar cheese.

Whole Grain Bread. Public eating places are most deficient in whole grain breads. Whole wheat sandwich bread is often available, but may not be entirely whole grain. Choose sourdough over others. Sourdough is usually easier to digest.

Chili and refried beans are good sources of fiber, but may be high in fat and too salty. Inquire. Request a sample. You can judge the fat and salt for yourself that way.

Save pasta dishes for home cooking when you can use whole grain pasta. When you have a choice between rice pilaf, baked potato, or mashed potatoes, take the baked potato. The rice is white and the mashed potatoes usually are from a box of potato flakes.

Baked Potato makes a good main dish. Learn to enjoy the skin! With a salad the baked potato can be a satisfying and totally nutritious main dish. It is not fattening and provides good protein (see below).

Low Fat

Topping for the Baked Potato: You can complement the protein by requesting a protein topping instead of the usual butter or margarine. Ask the waitress to give half sour cream blended with half lowfat cottage cheese or plain yogurt. Or you can take your little container of nonfat or lowfat yogurt from home and mix it with the sour cream. Put plenty on the potato to provide that pleasing contrast in hot and cold temperature and to moisten the potato so it isn't dry. A ¼ cup blend of lowfat yogurt and sour cream will provide 111 calories, 5.5 grams protein, and 8 grams fat. If you use lowfat cottage cheese in place of the sour cream you will have 95 calories, 10.5 grams of protein, and only 2.5 grams of fat! Quite an improvement over even one tablespoon of butter at 102 calories, with no protein and 12 grams of fat.

At the salad bar leave the prepared salads such as macaroni, potato, and coleslaw with lots of mayonnaise in them behind. Three-bean salad, well-drained, or pickled vegetables add tang without the fat.

Choose lemon juice, vinegar and olive oil, or cottage cheese as good salad toppings in place of oil dressings. If you use oil dressing, aim for one tablespoon well-distributed over the greenery.

Request salad dressings, gravies, and sauces to be served on the side. Let 1 tablespoon be your "measuring" guide.

Order meats that are baked or broiled, and unbreaded. Choose fish and chicken instead of beef. Request fish to be cooked without fat. Remove the skin from the chicken. Roast beef has less fat than hamburger.

If you don't order refined white flour rolls or bread you won't have a decision to make about using butter on them.

Ask for butter in place of margarine. This goes against what everyone else says to do (see p. 78). Limit yourself to one pat.

Main dishes with cheese sauce or cream sauce will be very high in fat. If you want one of these, order one dish for two people, eat a small portion, and fill up on the fresh salad.

Skip cakes, pies, quick breads, cream cheese, and ice cream desserts. Have fresh fruit, frozen yogurt, or a taste of someone else's dessert.

For children order water, real fruit juice, or nonfat milk to drink. Most children enjoy orange juice. Avoid homogenized milk (see p. 91).

Avoid deep-fat-fried foods such as French fries, fried chicken, fried shrimp, and scallops. You can take the skin off of fried chicken, however.

If you order a vegetarian hot dish, request that only a very small amount of fat, such as used in stir-fry, be used. Some places use a lot!

Choose clear soups with vegetables, chicken, or beef in preference to cream soups. Find out, however, if a lot of fat is in the broth and request "not salty." Ask for a taste first! Ask if it is homemade. They are usually better.

Not Too Much

This is more a matter of discipline and self-control. Some commitments made in advance will help. First, decide not to order a full dinner per person. Order salad or soup for each person and share a dinner between two people. Practically every restaurant dinner is big enough for two!

Tortilla chip appetizer in Mexican restaurants: Make a prior commitment to let the first bowlful suffice. If you like the appetizer "hot," order extra salsa and enjoy much "hot" with little chips.

Order soup and salad and nothing else. Wait until you have finished before ordering anything more. You probably won't want anything else!

Less Salt

Leave the salt shaker in its place on the table.

Request meats, fish, poultry to be cooked without salt.

Ask to taste the soup before ordering. Oversalting soups is a common practice. If enough customers ask about this, chefs will catch on.

Skip potato chips, French fries, breaded meats, and breaded fish.

Casserole dishes will be higher in salt than fresh salads and fruits.

Low Sweets

Order fresh fruit or frozen yogurt for dessert.

Skip dessert or have a taste of someone else's.

Don't order muffins, nut breads, cornbread, or quick breads, in general. These have more sugar in them than yeast breads such as dinner rolls, sandwich breads, and crusty French loaves. Almost all of them are made with white flour, anyway.

Natural Food Restaurants

Now you have the general guidelines. What are the best restaurants to look for? Natural food restaurants have much more to offer nutritionally than other restaurants. Usually you will have a good variety of whole grain breads, brown rice, and whole grain pasta dishes to choose from. There is more variety in the salad greenery and more opportunity to find dishes utilizing meats in smaller quantity. Sometimes vegetable oil can be overused. It is a good idea to ask about the amount used. Natural food restaurants offer greater variety of imaginative dishes utilizing fresh vegetables and fruits. Some vegetarian restaurants have an Eastern cultic atmosphere. If you take guests to one of these, make sure they will not feel uncomfortable there.

Ethnic Food

Ethnic foods often offer more nutrition than traditional American fare. Chinese restaurants offer more vegetables. You can ask for the MSG (monosodium glutamate) to be omitted. Oriental restaurants seldom serve brown rice. If you like Chinese food, ask for brown rice. If proprietors hear such requests from customers repeatedly, they will begin to catch on. Businesses want to please their customers. Repeat business means profit.

Many Japanese restaurants offer both plant and fish seafood, tofu, and many vegetables. Avoid the deep-fried foods, especially the shellfish. Sushi (raw fish wrapped in a variety of ingredients) is usually safe to eat.

Indian restaurants are not common, but Indian food offers some good choices, such as curry dishes and yogurt. Mexican food can be a better choice than standard American fast foods. Request corn tortillas that are not fried. They can be warmed without fat. Choose the dishes with lots of greenery.

Most Mexican food has more greenery and beans and less meat. The beans may contain lard, however. Go for the salad-type dishes in preference to ones with cheese.

What About Fast Foods?

Drive by them fast! The problem is not the "fast" but the food. Look for what isn't fried, what isn't refined, what isn't oversalted, and what isn't full of sugar. Some fastfood places are installing salad bars. Opt for the pizza parlor ahead of the hamburger, fried chicken, or fish 'n chips places. Although pizza is made with a white flour crust, there is a higher proportion of nonmeat goodies on top. Skip the pepperoni and try for plain cheese or the vegetable-topped choices. Order a small serving of pizza and take a big salad with it. Actually, if you really want a hamburger and have access to a natural foods restaurant, buy a hamburger there on a whole wheat bun with extra fresh ingredients.

Traveling by Air?

You can request three days ahead for special meals on most airlines. Your travel agent can also do this for you. Emilie does this often. She has received beautiful salads, vegetable meals, pasta, and fruit platters. Remember that good business is serving the customer's wishes!

Traveling by Car?

As long-distance travelers, Rich and Sue have developed a system for eating out that is enjoyable and uncomplicated. They carry granola and buy fresh fruit, yogurt, and skim milk along the way for breakfasts. For lunches they buy leafy lettuce, a tomato, cheddar cheese, Hollywood mayonnaise, carrots, a couple pieces of fresh fruit, and real fruit juice. At a rest stop they prepare a vegetable salad or sandwiches (if whole wheat bread is available). For dinner they eat out following the guidelines listed. The food expense is very low.

Eating out costs twice as much as eating the same meal at home.

When Rich and Sue traveled to Mexico City by train, granola, yogurt, fresh fruit purchased along the way, and their own water supply were sustaining and satisfying.

Eating with Friends

It won't be long before your friends realize that you like healthy food. In the meantime, offer to bring one of the dishes. You can't go wrong by offering to bring the salad, some muffins, or the dessert. This gives you opportunity to introduce whole foods in a winsome way. You don't have to make any comments about what you bring or what you are served. Eat smaller amounts of the less-nutritious items and larger amounts of the more-nutritious. Thank your host and hostess for their hospitality. Don't discuss nutrition unless you are invited to answer some questions or inquiries.

If you know your conscience will bother you if you eat a certain food such as pork, let your hostess know in advance that you do not eat that food. This need not be offensive. What is offensive is passing judgment, showing disdain, or rejecting food when it is set in front of you. If you have a health problem such as allergies, your hostess will be only too glad to omit it from the menu if you inform her in advance.

Potlucks and Smorgasbords

These occasions are temptations to gorge, so you'll need to exercise a little restraint. Usually there is a wide enough variety to find some nutritious selections. Sue always takes a big fresh salad and whole grain muffins or rolls so that there are at least two nutritious items. Eating at a potluck is not the same as eating with friends in their home. People usually don't pay much attention to whose dishes you eat or what you eat at a potluck.

Breakfast Out?

Fresh fruit, real fruit juice, hot or cold cereal, whole wheat toast with butter and/or honey, decaffeinated coffee or tea, and egg omelets that aren't too cheesy, or poached eggs are good choices. Avoid the pancakes, waffles, French toast, and muffins unless they are whole grain. Omit the bacon and pork sausage. If you desire meat, ask for a small lean beef patty in place of the pork. If you like potatoes, request that they be fried in one tablespoon or less of fat.

A Few Extras

Peppermint or spearmint tea sipped slowly with the meal will assist in digestion of the food. Take your own tea bags and ask for hot water.

Meats eaten after salads may hinder digestion. Eat the meat with the salad.

Let the establishment know that you appreciate choices. Some restaurants request written evaluations. Be sure to write on it that you would like the option to order whole grain bread or rolls and brown rice.

In lieu of sour cream request a blend of sour cream and nonfat or lowfat yogurt. Again, if proprietors get requests often enough, they will begin to oblige. Tradition fogs imagination. Some things, such as keeping yogurt on hand, would be such an easy thing to do.

Request purified or bottled water. You can also request fresh lemon to squeeze into it.

Remember, you are in control! Ask for exactly what you want even if you know the establishment doesn't have it. Consumer demand is what elicits change in our profit oriented society.

53

Food Storage and Safety Tips

- Make sure your refrigerator is 40° or less and your freezer zero degrees or less.
- After opening, refrigerate wheat germ, pure maple syrup, vegetable oils, salad dressings, mayonnaise, jams, jellies, peanut butter without sugar or hydrogenated fat added, and shelled nuts.
- Store shelled nuts, sunflower seeds, and sesame seeds purchased in quantity in the freezer.
- Uncooked bulgur (parboiled wheat) does not require refrigeration even during the hot days of summer. Neither does white rice. Brown rice also keeps well unrefrigerated for a month, and refrigerated for six months.
- When you store basic ingredients such as canned broth or tomatoes, rotate the older containers to the front of your cupboard or refrigerator or date them with a marking pen to use first.
- To prevent contamination of food inside containers, always use a clean utensil to scoop out mayonnaise, peanut butter, tomato paste, etc. Never eat directly from the container except for one taste with a clean utensil.
- To reduce contact with air which may cause food to deteriorate more quickly, store foods and leftovers in the smallest possible containers. This also gives you more room in the refrigerator.
- In warm weather, unless your kitchen is air-conditioned, consider storing whole grain flours, crackers and breads in the refrigerator or freezer, unless you can use them quickly. Refrigeration tends to dry out breads. Slice loaves first and freeze them unless they are to be eaten within three or four days.

- Wholegrain crackers with no preservatives added go rancid quickly. Store in refrigerator or freezer if not used up in a couple of weeks.
- To keep crackers crisp, store them in a canister with a dry paper towel inside the cover. To recrisp soft crackers, place them on a cookie sheet in a 250° oven for about 10 minutes.
- Honey keeps best in a warm, dark place. It will crystallize in the refrigerator making it inconvenient to use. Warm crystallized honey over low heat in a pan of water to reliquefy it.
- We love raisins that are soft and chewy in cereal. Buy cold cereals plain and a large package of raisins. Pour ½ cup boiling water over the raisins in a jar, cover tightly with a lid and shake up a bit. Let cool and refrigerate until cereal time. Take out as many as needed.
- When using a grater, put masking tape or a bandage on your thumb. It works every time—and no more hurt thumb.
- Frozen foods have a definite freezer life. Use food within the specified period of time. Meats, such as ground beef, turkey, and franks keep 2-3 months, roast beef up to 12 months. Wrap properly in freezer wrap. Wax paper won't do. Sandwich meats keep only one month. Mark packages with "USE BY" date. Your market does this, and it makes good sense.

Useful Leftovers

- Chop small amounts of leftover cooked turkey, chicken, or beef into chunks for adding to soup, a hearty main dish, chili, or spaghetti.
- Freeze the few extra tablespoons of fruit juice left in the bottom of the bottle in an ice cube tray. Pop the cubes into a plastic bag to store until you roast a turkey or chicken. Perfect for basting!
- Put leftover rice in a greased casserole and cover with home-made cheese sauce. Sprinkle with grated cheese and bake at 350° for 20 minutes or use leftover rice in stuffing as a substitute for bread. Also great for putting into soups or making rice pudding.

- Save leftover pancakes or waffles. Pop them into the toaster or oven for a quick, easy breakfast or after-school snack. Waffles also reheat perfectly in the waffle iron set at medium temperature.
- Keep a leftover list on the refrigerator with date stored and what container item is stored in. Write item on menu where you can use it up.

Timesaver Tips

- Make your own convenience foods. Chop large batches of onion, green pepper, or nuts and freeze in small units. Grate a week's or month's worth of cheese and freeze it in recipe-size portions. Shape ground meat or ground turkey into patties so you can thaw a few at a time. Freeze home-made casseroles, soups, stews, and chili in serving-size portions for faster thawing and reheating. Menu planning will help you take advantage of doing these things!
- Leave bread "rejects" in a basket to dry in the open air. When you have several slices, make crumbs with them in the blender and freeze in a tightly covered Tupperware container or a plastic bag. They'll be ready to use when you need them.
- To speed up baking potatoes, put a clean nail through the potato and it will bake in half the time.
- For quick, easy cleanup when preparing sticky hot cereal or steaming rice, coat the inside of the saucepan with vegetable cooking spray beforehand. Try it also on the blades of the food processor when mixing dough.
- When measuring oil and honey, measure the oil before the honey. The honey will pour right out of the oiled measuring cup.
- Keep a grocery list on your refrigerator or bulletin board and write down each item when you notice that you need to restock. By the time you are ready to shop, all the "extras" that you might otherwise forget are already listed.
- Make cleanup after each food preparation part of the preparation. Clutter from the last task will not be in your way and by mealtime your kitchen will be clean.

Utensils and Equipment for the Kitchen

Here is a list of basics you should have when cooking:

Liquid measuring cups—2 cup measure will handle many jobs.

Dry measuring cups—These usually come in nested sets from ¼ to 1 cup.

Measuring spoons—These also come in sets which include ¼ teaspoon, ½ teaspoon, 1 teaspoon and 1 tablespoon.

Wooden spoons and large metal spoons—A cook should have several of each kind. A slotted spoon is also useful.

Rubber spatulas—You should have at least one wide one; a narrow rubber spatula is useful for scraping out jars and small bowls.

Wire Whisk—A wire whisk at least as long as a rubber scraper will perform many important hand blending jobs.

Shredder—One with fine holes for grating things such as lemon peel; another with larger holes for grating cheese, cabbage, and carrots.

Timer—Most stoves have timers, but if yours does not work, there are hand-held timers that are very accurate.

Tongs—To lift things out of water.

Colander—For draining things like spaghetti.

Rolling pin—An essential if you're going to make pastry.

Saucepans—The rule is to buy the best you can afford. A good, strong pan with a riveted handle and thick bottom will last a lifetime. It's nice to have a 1-quart, 2-quart, and 3-quart saucepan. But if you can only choose one, select a good 2-quart saucepan. Consider stainless steel waterless.

Dutch oven—This comes in handy for making such things as stews and sauces. It can also be used in the oven.

Skillet—A large frying pan with a lid is used in many different kinds of recipes. Cast iron lasts forever. Non-stick pans allow frying without fat or oil, but you can "saute" with a little water in any frying pan. To season a new cast iron pan, wash it with warm water and dry well. Put over a very hot burner, add a few tablespoons peanut oil and swirl it around the pan. Pour out the oil, cool the pan, and repeat the process. Food will not stick to a properly seasoned pan.

Baking pans—Those that are used frequently are an 8-inch square pan, a flat cookie sheet, 10 x 15 inch rimmed pan (jellyroll pan), 9 x 5 inch baking pan, 9-inch round cake pan, muffin pan, 9 x 5 inch loaf pan. A bundt pan is nice to have for baking whole grain cakes.

Wire racks—For cooling cookies, cakes, breads.

Knives—A good knife is worth its weight in gold. It can make cooking tasks so much easier. You should have a paring knife, French knife and a serrated bread knife. A chef's knife makes wonderfully light work of chopping nuts, dried fruits, and vegetables. A steel to sharpen the knives is essential.

Electric Mixer—There are many different kinds. Even small, hand-held ones make cooking tasks easier.

Blender—Indispensable to whole foods preparation. One that will crack ice, make bread crumbs, chop nuts, and mince parsley will do almost anything else you'll need.

Wok—Makes quick, light work of stir-frying, especially a non-stick electric one. Also useful for steaming large amounts of food such as big pieces of squash or pumpkin, a large bunch of dark leafy greens.

Waffle Iron—a nice, but not necessary, appliance for making delicious whole grain waffles!

54

How to Read a Label

Advertising Slogans

Food companies thrive on the nutritional half-truth that will sell the product. These selling points are printed in large letters on the front of the package. Do not buy a product merely because one of the following terms appears on the front: no preservatives added, all-natural, 100% natural, no sugar added, low calorie, low fat, no salt added, low cholesterol. These facts may be important, but you'll want to know much more. For example, many products without preservatives are refined carbohydrates containing mostly white flour and white sugar. Any product can be labeled natural and contain white flour and white sugar since both ingredients are food. Find out all the ingredients in the product.

The Ingredients List (The Best Guide to Quality)

The most important part of the label is the ingredients list in fine print on the back, side, or end of the container. Ingredients are listed in descending amounts by weight. The first listed ingredient is the most by weight in the product. Watch for several different kinds of sugars listed. If there are two or three kinds, there may be more sugar in the product than the first named ingredient. For example: "wheat flour, brown sugar, soybean oil, honey, yeast, salt."

Ingredients to avoid are: hydrogenated fat or vegetable oil, partially hydrogenated fat or vegetable oils, shortening, refined sugars such as high fructose corn syrup, corn syrup solids, sucrose, dextrose, sugar, brown sugar, wheat flour (it is white unless designated whole wheat), enriched white or wheat flour, bleached enriched white flour, degerminated cornmeal.

215

There are thousands of additives, with new ones emerging daily. To know about every one is impossible. More important is that the products containing additives seldom include whole food ingredients as the primary ingredients. If the product does not contain real whole food ingredients, it isn't nutritionally worth buying anyway. Avoid artificial flavorings, colorings, sodium nitrite and nitrate, sodium bisulfite, and saccharin. The cumulative effects of preservatives on the human body are not known. Although you should read labels in every store, you will have a much easier time finding prepackaged convenience foods without additives in health food stores. A helpful reference to additives is *What's That You're Eating?!!* by C. D. King.

The Nutrient Data

Many package labels list nutrient data such as grams of protein, fat, carbohydrate, sodium, and fiber. Vitamins and minerals are seldom listed unless added synthetically. Often a percentage of the RDA's for a few nutrients are given, but this information is not too useful. It is difficult to assess true nutritional value by the nutrient data. Nutrient data may be given for a serving size that is much different than a normal serving. If you look at nutrient data only, it is difficult to distinguish a refined from a whole food product. The ingredients label is a better guide. The most useful nutrient data is the amount of sodium and dietary fiber. Few food packages currently include dietary fiber. If the label lists crude fiber, it is not a useful measure. Fat percentage is usually listed by weight, not by calories. It is percentage by calories that gives you a true measure for staying within the 30% recommended daily limit.

A Comparison

Read the labels of the following two products. Both are the same food item. Which one would you buy? Note that the ingredients lists are a much better guide to quality than the nutrient data.

1 *Ingredients*: 100% whole wheat flour, amaranth flour, pure honey, unsulphured molasses, graham flour, soybean oil, baking soda, lecithin, salt

Nutrient data (1 serving): 60 calories, 1 gram protein, 1 gram fat, 11 grams carbohydrate, 45 mg. sodium, 35 mg. potassium

2 *Ingredients*: enriched wheat flour (containing niacin, reduced iron, thiamine mononitrate and riboflavin), sugar, graham flour, partially hydrogenated vegetable shortening (contains one or more of the following: soybean oil, coconut oil, palm oil, cottonseed oil), brown sugar, corn syrup, honey, sodium bicarbonate, salt, molasses, lecithin, malted cereal syrup and vanillin

Nutrient data (1 serving): 60 calories, 1 gram protein, 2 grams fat, 11 grams carbohydrate, 50 mg. sodium, 20 mg. potassium

55

How to Locate Shopping Resources

Look in the yellow pages of your phone book under the following topics. These can lead you to other resources. Call companies on the phone and ask questions that concern you—Do you market organic or organic certified products? Do you mail order? Do you order or sell in bulk? Can you refer me to someone who sells (name of item/s)?

Bakers
Beans—Dried
Cookware
Dehydrating Equipment
Eggs
Fish
Flea Markets
Flour Dealers
Food Products
Foods, Dehydrated and Freeze-Dried
Fruits and Vegetables
Grain Dealers
Health
Herbs
Honey
Magic Mill & Mixer (look in white pages)
Meat
Milk
Nuts
Poultry
Spices
Vitamins and Food Supplements

Friends are often the best leads to unique local resources such as food co-ops, offerings of local farmers and bee-keepers, produce stands or shops, flea markets, etc.

MAIL ORDER SOURCES

Send for catalog, price list, and shipping information from any of the sources listed on the following page.

The Meat Shop
6522 Fremont N.
Seattle, WA 98103
(206) 783-5751

Certified organic, no
hormones or antibiotics.
Chickens, turkey, Shelton
frozen poultry, fresh fish,
beef, lamb, veal, packaged
meats without nitrates or
nitrites, MSG, or other
preservatives.

Walnut Acres
Penns Creek, PA 17862
24 Hour Credit Card Line:
(717) 837-0601

Organic, chemical free, and
nonorganic. Complete line
of whole food products,
family-size packages.

**Mountain Ark Trading
Company**
120 South East Avenue
Fayettville, AR 72701
(800) 643-8909

Many organic. Complete
line of staple whole food
products. Specializes in
macrobiotic foods—miso,
sea vegetables, etc.

Pine Ridge Farms
P.O. Box 98
Subiaco, AR 72865
(501) 934-4565

Certified organic. Chickens,
turkey, ground turkey.

Oak Manor Farms
R.R. 1 Tavistock
Ontario, Canada
NOB 2RO
(519) 662-2385

Certified organic. Grains,
flours, seeds, cereals, no-
salt chips, pastas, nuts,
dried fruits, carob chips/
powder, yeast, baking
powder.

American Orsa Salt, Inc.
75 North State Street
Redmond, UT 84652
(801) 529-3526

Unheated Natural Mineral
Salt—2, 5, 25, or 50 pounds.

**Giusto's Specialty Foods,
Inc.**
241 East Harris Avenue
South San Francisco, CA
94080

Organic. Beans, grains,
flours, flakes, cereals, oils,
seeds, spices, baking
powder, oils, sea salt.

Deer Valley Farm
R.D. 1
Guilford, NY 13780
(607) 794-8556

Organic. Complete line of staple whole foods. Beef, lamb, fish, ground turkey, Dr. Bronner's Balanced Protein Seasoning (same as Bernard Jensen's Natural Vegetable Seasoning).

Arrowhead Mills, Inc.
P.O. Box 2059
Hereford, TX 79045

Organic. Grains, cereals, flakes, beans, nuts, seeds, dried fruits and vegetables.

Shelton Farms
204 N. Lorraine
Pomona, CA 91767
(714) 623-4361

Organic. Chickens, turkey, ground turkey, chicken and turkey pot pies, turkey sausage links.

Jaffe Bros.
P.O. Box 636
Valley Center, CA 92082-0636
(619) 749-1133

Organic. Dried fruits, nuts/ butters, grains, pastas, seeds, beans, honey, carob, coconut, oil, olives, peas and beans, mushrooms, pickles, relish.

Flour Mills and Bread Kneaders
Eating Better Newsletter
8830 Glencoe Drive
Riverside, CA 92503

Request: Equipment Reviews and Sources.

Garden Spot Distributors
Rt. 1, Box 729A
New Holland, PA 17557
(800) 292-9631 in
    Pennsylvania
(800) 445-5100 in
    Northeast
(717) 354-4936 in
    other areas

Organic. Full line of products. Specialize in frozen. Poultry, meat, ground turkey.

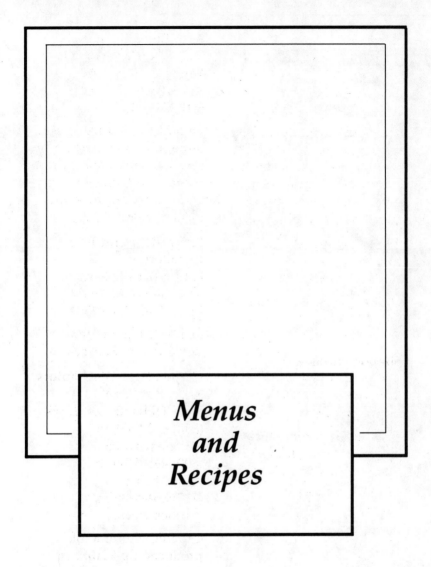

*Menus
and
Recipes*

Unlimited Menu Plan

SUN	MON	TUES	WED	THURS	FRI	SAT
Tamale Pie Fiesta (p. 235)	Veggie Burrito King (p. 241)	Yams in Orange Sauce or Baked Yam (p. 231)	Kid's Choice	Lemon Baked Fish (p. 258)	Split Pea Soup (p. 242)	Fettuccine (p. 255)
Fruit Bowl Meal	Ratatouille over Baked Potato (p. 247)	Chicken Chop Suey (p. 262)	Little Cottage Enchiladas (p. 254)	Middle Eastern Lentil Soup (p. 243)	Almond Tuna Salad (p. 266)	Sweet 'n Sour Tofu Stir-fry (p. 249)
Turkey Burgers (pp. 236-37)	Brown Rice Pilaf with Mexi-Salad (p. 227)	Eggplant Parmigiana (p. 239)	Golden Stuffed Potatoes (p. 232)	Dad's Choice	Cashew Chicken (p. 261)	Creole Black-eyed Peas 'n Corn (p. 246)
Zucchini Sausage Bake (p. 238)	Barley Casserole (p. 229)	Baked Salmon (p. 259)	Saucy Spaghetti (p. 240)	Lentil Rice Casserole (p. 228)	Dine Out	Marinated Tofu Stir-fry (p. 252)
Vegetable Lasagna (p. 248)	Golden Waffles or Pancakes (p. 233)	Baked Parmesan Chicken (p. 260)	Dinner with Bob and Emilie	Chili or Savory Chili (pp. 244-45)	Tuna Noodle Yummy (p. 256)	Leftover "Potluck"

No Meat Menu Plan (Lacto-Vegetarian)
(meats, fish, poultry excluded)

SUN	MON	TUES	WED	THURS	FRI	SAT
				Creole Black-eyed Peas 'n Corn (p. 246)	Brown Rice Pilaf with Mexi-Salad (p. 227)	Dine Out
Split Pea Soup (p. 242)	Saucy Spaghetti Parmesan (p. 240)	Kid's Choice	Little Cottage Enchiladas (p. 254)	Yams in Orange Sauce or Baked Yam (p. 230)	Savory Leftovers	Cashew Chop Suey (p. 263)
Chili or Savory Chili (pp. 244-45)	Dinner with Rich and Sue	Sweet 'n Sour Tofu Stir-fry (p. 249)	Veggie Burrito King (p. 241)	Dad's Choice	Golden Waffles or Pancakes (p. 233)	Eggplant Parmigiana (p. 239)
Fruit Bowl Meal	Golden Stuffed Potatoes (p. 232)	Fettuccine (p. 255)				

No Dairy - No Egg Menu Plan

SUN	MON	TUES	WED	THURS	FRI	SAT
				Marinated Tofu Stir-fry (p. 252)	Turkey Burgers (pp. 236-37)	Dine Out
Chili or Savory Chili (pp. 244-45)	Brown Rice Pilaf with Mexi-Salad (p. 227)	Kid's Choice	Middle Eastern Lentil Soup (p. 243)	Lemon Baked Fish (p. 258)	Savory Leftovers	Ratatouille over Baked Potato (p. 247)
Split Pea Soup (p. 242)	Dinner with Bob and Emilie	Almond Tuna Salad (p. 266)	Saucy Spaghetti (p. 240)	Dad's Choice	Golden Stuffed Potatoes (p. 232)	Creole Black-eyed Peas 'n Corn (p. 246)
Fruit Bowl Meal	Chicken Chop Suey (p. 262)	Yams in Orange Sauce or Baked Yam (p. 230)				

BROWN RICE
3 Cups — 4 to 6 Servings

Place in saucepan and bring to a boil:
2 to 2½ cups water
1 cup brown rice, washed
1 teaspoon salt

Boil uncovered for 5 minutes.

Lower heat to very low, cover with a tight-fitting lid and simmer 45 to 60 minutes.

Do not uncover during cooking! Do not stir during cooking! Can develop sticky rice.

½-cup serving long-grain:
111 calories, 2.5 grams protein, 23 grams carbohydrate, 0.5 grams fat (6% of calories), 2 grams dietary fiber

Nutrient data on all recipes rounded off to nearest whole or half gram.

BROWN RICE PILAF
6 Servings

Combine together in saucepan:
1½ cups uncooked long-grain brown rice
¼ cup chopped almonds
3 cups chicken broth
2 teaspoons soy sauce
⅛ teaspoon garlic powder

Bring to a boil and boil uncovered for 5 minutes.

Cover with tight-fitting lid, reduce heat to low and simmer 50 to 60 minutes or until all the water is absorbed. Do not remove lid during cooking and do not stir (may cause sticky rice).

While rice cooks, sauté for 1 to 2 minutes in 2 or 3 tablespoons water:
2 green onions, chopped

Fold onions into cooked rice just before serving.

VARIATION:
—In place of chicken broth use 3 cups water with 4 teaspoons Bernard Jensen's Natural Vegetable Seasoning (see Shopping Guide, p. 196).

Serve with:
Broccoli (pp. 264-65)
Mexi-Salad (tossed salad with added kidney beans, garbanzo beans, grated cheese, if desired)

1 serving long-grain:
204 calories, 5.5 grams protein, 37 grams carbohydrate, 4 grams fat (17% of calories), 2 grams dietary fiber

LENTIL RICE CASSEROLE
6 Servings

Blend together in a casserole dish:
3 cups chicken broth
³/₄ cup lentils, uncooked
¹/₂ cup brown rice, uncooked
¹/₄ cup instant minced onion (or ³/₄ cup fresh chopped)
¹/₂ teaspoon sweet basil
¹/₄ teaspoon oregano
¹/₄ teaspoon thyme
¹/₄ teaspoon garlic powder

Bake covered for 2 to 2¹/₂ hours at 300°.

During last 20 minutes of baking top with:
¹/₂ cup grated cheddar cheese (optional)

Just before serving, stir to blend in the melted cheese and garnish with:
a handful of minced fresh parsley

VARIATION:
—In place of chicken broth use water and 1 tablespoon Bernard Jensen's Natural Vegetable Seasoning (see Shopping Guide, p. 196).

Serve with:
Plain yogurt or barbecue sauce
Green or yellow vegetable
Tossed salad or lettuce-orange-pineapple salad

1 serving without cheese:
155 calories, 9.5 grams protein, 29 grams carbohydrate, 0.5 grams fat (4% of calories), 3.5 grams dietary fiber

1 serving with cheese:
193 calories, 10.5 grams protein, 29 grams carbohydrate, 3.5 grams fat (17% of calories), 3.5 grams dietary fiber

BARLEY CASSEROLE
6 Servings

Brown over medium heat, stirring frequently for about 10 minutes:
> ³/₄ **cup pearled barley, uncooked**

Lightly sauté in 2 or 3 tablespoons water:
> **¹/₂ onion, chopped**
> **1 stalk celery, chopped**
> **1 small green pepper, chopped**

Bring to a boil in a saucepan:
> **2 cups chicken or beef broth**
> **2 teaspoons soy sauce**

Pour hot broth into 9" x 13" pan or casserole and mix in:
> **browned barley**
> **sautéed vegetables**
> **2 oz. (¹/₄ cup) mushroom stems and pieces, drained**
> **small (8³/₄ oz.) can garbanzo beans, drained**
> **¹/₂ of an 8-oz. can water chestnuts, sliced and drained**

Cover and bake at 350° for 1¹/₂ to 2 hours until barley is tender and liquid is absorbed.

VARIATION:
—Add 1¹/₂ teaspoons Bernard Jensen's Natural Vegetable Seasoning (see Shopping Guide, p. 196).

Serve with:
Green or yellow vegetable
Tossed salad

1 serving:
161 calories, 6 grams protein, 33 grams carbohydrate, 0.5 grams fat (3% of calories), 3.5 grams dietary fiber

YAMS IN ORANGE SAUCE
6 to 8 Servings

Bake at 375° about 45 minutes until almost tender:
   6 medium yams or sweet potatoes

Peel and slice yams into lightly buttered casserole dish.

Blend together and pour over top of yams:
   1 cup orange juice
   ¼ cup honey or fructose, granulated
   2 tablespoons melted butter
   2 tablespoons arrowroot powder or cornstarch

Cover and bake at 350° for 30 minutes.

VARIATIONS:
—Add a cup or two of small fresh pineapple chunks.
—Top with a few chopped dates and cinnamon.

Serve with:
Green vegetable
Waldorf salad
Whole grain muffins or bread

1 serving (when 6 servings made):
347 calories, 4 grams protein, 74 grams carbohydrate, 5 grams fat (13% of calories), 5 grams dietary fiber.

BAKED YAM OR SWEET POTATO

Yams sold in the U.S. are a variety of sweet potato. A true yam is very low in nutrients while 1 cup of mashed sweet potato contains 20,000 IU's provitamin A, 43 mg. vitamin C, 82 mg. calcium, and 620 mg. potassium.

Scrub and bake at 400° about 1 hour or until done:
1 baking potato (about 8 oz.) per person

Eat the skins, just like Irish skins!

1 serving (8-oz. potato):

322 calories, 5 grams protein, 74 grams carbohydrate, 1 gram fat (3% of calories), 9 grams dietary fiber.

GOLDEN STUFFED POTATOES
4 Servings

A tasty alternative to butter-laden potatoes! These make a big hit when served to company. Serve with no extra butter at the table.

Wash and bake at 400° until done, about 1 hour:
3 baking size (8 oz.) potatoes

Meanwhile cut into about 3" chunks:
**about 1 lb. banana or yellow squash, seeds removed—
to make 1¼ cups mashed cooked squash**

Place squash skin side down in vegetable steamer over boiling water, cover, and steam until very tender, about 20 to 30 minutes. Add more water, if needed.

When squash is cooled off enough to handle (but still very warm), scoop squash from skin with a spoon into electric mixer bowl (if you have one—otherwise into regular mixing bowl).

When baked potatoes are cool enough to handle (but still hot), cut in half lengthwise and scoop potato with spoon into bowl with the squash.

Add:
1 tablespoon soft butter
1 teaspoon salt
³⁄₈ to ½ teaspoon cumin powder, to taste

Blend until smooth with electric beaters or potato masher. Pile potato-squash mixture into potato shells. Garnish with paprika. Place in covered pan or casserole and return to oven to heat through.

Serve with:
Amandine green beans or green vegetable
Apple coleslaw
Minute Bran or Whole Grain Muffins (p. 270).

1 serving:
113 calories, 2.5 grams protein, 19 grams carbohydrate, 3 grams fat (25% of calories), 4 grams dietary fiber

GOLDEN WAFFLES/PANCAKES
4 to 6 Servings

An easy dinner! Makes 3 to 4 large waffles or about 20 pancakes.

Blend together dry ingredients:
1½ cups whole wheat flour
1½ cups stoneground cornmeal
1 tablespoon baking powder
1 teaspoon salt

Mix into dry ingredients:
4 eggs
2½ cups buttermilk, as needed for consistency

Spray hot waffle iron or pancake griddle well with Pam spray or add 1 tablespoon melted butter or oil to batter to prevent sticking.

VARIATIONS:
—For lighter waffles or pancakes, separate the eggs, beat egg whites until stiff, but not dry, and fold into batter last.

—Add chopped nuts to batter or sprinkle over top of each waffle just before closing waffle iron lid to bake. Pecans or sunflower seeds are good.

—Add 2 to 4 tablespoons melted butter or vegetable oil for a more delectable texture.

Serve with:
Unsweetened applesauce and/or pure maple syrup or fresh strawberries
Lowfat vanilla or plain yogurt

1 serving (when 6 servings made)—added fat not included:

317 calories, 14.5 grams protein, 50 grams carbohydrate, 7 grams fat (20% of calories), 7.5 grams dietary fiber

SEASONED GROUND TURKEY
1 Pound

Great for using in any recipe calling for hamburger or ground beef; seasoning really improves flavor!

Mix thoroughly and brown in frying pan:
  1 lb. ground turkey
  ⅛ teaspoon nutmeg
  ⅛ teaspoon thyme
  ⅛ teaspoon garlic powder
  ⅛ teaspoon sage
  1 tablespoon soy sauce
  2 tablespoons tomato sauce or ketchup

TAMALE PIE FIESTA
6 Servings

Season and brown:
   1 lb. ground turkey (p. 234)

When turkey is about half-browned, add and saute until turkey is cooked:
   1 small green pepper, chopped
   1 small onion, chopped
   1 clove garlic, minced

Lower heat and blend in:
   2 cups tomato sauce
   2 cups corn, frozen or fresh
   2¹/₄ oz. sliced ripe olives, drained (optional)
   1¹/₂ teaspoons chili powder
   ¹/₂ teaspoon salt

When hot remove from heat and pour into 9" square baking pan, small 9" x 13" baking pan, or 2-quart casserole dish.

In saucepan bring to boil:
   1 cup water
   ¹/₂ teaspooon salt
   1 tablespoon butter

In separate bowl blend cornmeal into a second cup of water:
   1 cup cold water
   1 cup stoneground cornmeal

Gradually stir cold water-cornmeal mixture into boiling water, stirring to thicken, about 2 minutes. Spread cooked cornmeal mixture evenly to edges over top of casserole.

Bake uncovered for 40 to 50 minutes at 350°.

Serve with:
Green vegetable
Tossed salad

1 serving (includes olives):

197 calories, 19 grams protein, 33 grams carbohydrate, 14.5 grams fat (66% of calories), 7 grams dietary fiber

TURKEY BURGER PATTIES
4 Patties

A tasty alternative to hamburger patties, lower in fat and calories!

Mix together:
1 lb. ground turkey
seasonings for Seasoned Ground Turkey (p. 234)

Shape 4 burger patties.
Bake in oven at 350° for 10 to 15 minutes in shallow pan. May also be fried, but not as moist this way. No fat is needed to cook turkey burger in any pan.

To barbecue, set patties in foil cupped around the edges; otherwise meat will fall through grill.

1 patty:

216 calories, 20.5 grams protein, 1 gram carbohydrate, 15 grams fat (63% of calories), no fiber

TURKEY BURGER
1 Serving

> **Whole wheat hamburger bun or bread**
> **2 tablespoons Thousand Island Dressing** (p. 278)
> **Turkey Burger Patty** (p. 236)
> **1 thick slice tomato**
> **1 slice onion**
> **¼ cup alfalfa sprouts**
> **leafy green lettuce leaves**

Serve with:
Carrot and celery sticks, cucumber slices

1 burger:
551 calories, 32.5 grams protein, 42 grams carbohydrate, 27 grams fat (44% of calories), 5.5 grams dietary fiber

ZUCCHINI SAUSAGE BAKE
6 Servings

In large frying pan or wok lightly brown zucchini in oil, remove from heat, drain, and set aside:
  2 tablespoons olive oil
  4 generous cups unpeeled zucchini slices (not too thin, not too thick)

Brown in same pan:
  1 chopped onion

While onion starts browning mix together:
  1 lb. ground turkey
  1 teaspoon salt
  1/2 teaspoon nutmeg
  1/2 teaspoon sage
  1/2 teaspoon thyme
  1/16 teaspoon cayenne pepper

Add ground turkey to onion and continue cooking until turkey is well browned; cool slightly. Meanwhile, measure into a bowl:
  2 cups lowfat milk

Heat 1³/₄ cup of the milk. To the remaining ¹/₄ cup milk blend in:
  2 tablespoons arrowroot powder or cornstarch

Blend arrowroot or cornstarch-milk mixture into the hot milk, stirring constantly until thickened. Stir in:
  1 cup grated cheddar cheese

Blend together in mixing bowl:
  3 eggs, beaten
  1 cup whole wheat bread crumbs
  1 tablespoon minced fresh parsley
  1/8 teaspoon garlic powder
  browned turkey and onion

Layer cheese mixture, zucchini slices, and turkey mixture in a 2-qt. casserole, beginning and ending with sauce. Garnish with parsley, cover, and bake at 350° for 30 minutes.

Serve with:
Carrot salad
Whole grain muffins

1 serving:
405 calories, 27.5 grams protein, 14 grams carbohydrate, 27 grams fat (60% of calories), 5 grams dietary fiber

EGGPLANT PARMIGIANA
6 Servings

Beat lightly with a fork in a wide, shallow bowl:
2 eggs

Place in another wide, shallow bowl:
1 cup stoneground cornmeal, as needed

Thinly slice into ⅛"-thick slices:
1 medium eggplant, unpeeled

Dip eggplant slices first in eggs, then in cornmeal. Brown lightly in:
olive oil, as needed

Drain slices well on paper towels.

While slices are browning assemble:
2 8-oz. cans tomato sauce
2 cups mozzarella cheese, grated
¼ cup grated Parmesan cheese
2 teaspoons sweet basil

Make 2 or 3 layers of the ingredients in a lightly greased 9" x 13" pan in the following order:
eggplant slices
sauce
cheeses
sweet basil

Cover and bake at 350° for about 20 minutes or until cheese melts and sauce is heated through.

Serve with:
Green vegetable
Carrots, cabbage, or tossed salad

1 serving (using ¼ cup oil):
346 calories, 18 grams protein, 26 grams carbohydrate, 19.5 grams fat (51% of calories), 4.5 grams dietary fiber

SAUCY SPAGHETTI
6 Servings

Sauté in a little olive oil, or simmer in a little water for 5 to 10 minutes:
> **1 green pepper, chopped**
> **1 onion, chopped**
> **2 cloves garlic, minced**
> **1 cup fresh mushrooms, sliced,**
> > **or 4-oz. can stems and pieces**

Combine with sautéed vegetables in saucepan and simmer 30 minutes to blend flavors:
> **29-oz. can whole tomatoes, broken up**
> > **or two 12-oz. cans tomato sauce**
> **6-oz. can tomato paste**
> **1 teaspoon Italian seasoning, to taste**
> > **or: 1¼ teaspoon oregano**
> > **1¼ teaspoon sweet basil**
> > **1 teaspoon salt**
> > **¼ teaspoon thyme**
> > **⅛ teaspoon garlic powder**
> > **1 teaspoon soy sauce**

Meanwhile bring 4 quarts water to a boil, add spaghetti, and cook 10-15 minutes just until tender:
> **8-oz. package whole wheat spaghetti**
> **1 teaspoon olive oil**
> **¼ teaspoon salt**

Serve sauce over spaghetti. Top with Parmesan cheese, if desired.

VARIATION:
—Season 1 lb. ground turkey (p. 234) and add to spaghetti sauce.

Serve with:
Green or yellow vegetable
Tossed salad

---

1 serving (oil and cheese not included):

172 calories, 9 grams protein, 38 grams carbohydrate, 1.5 grams fat (8% of calories), 5 grams dietary fiber

VEGGIE BURRITO KING

There are no exact measurements for this sandwich. Mix together:
grated zucchini, unpeeled
grated carrot
chopped onion or chopped green onion

Add any or all of these optional ingredients:
grated cheddar cheese
shredded red cabbage
steamed broccoli and/or cauliflower pieces (cut small)
chopped green pepper
minced parsley
diced dill pickles

Season with your choice of:
cumin powder and sweet basil
and/or diced chilies and salsa
or Spike seasoning and barbecue sauce

Sauté filling in a little oil (preferably olive oil), if desired. Add any cheese after this, however. Have ready:
whole wheat tortillas or chapatis
yogurt or sour cream (one or the other, or half of each)

Place filling and yogurt-sour cream in center of tortillas and fold up. Wrap securely in foil and heat through thoroughly in oven at 350° about 20 minutes. Remove from foil and serve with the following on the side, as desired:
shredded lettuce
mound of alfalfa sprouts
chunks of avocado
tomato slices or wedges

Serve with:
Potato or mushroom soup
Fresh pineapple spears

1 burrito with 3 tablespoons cheese (estimate):
278 calories, 13 grams protein, 31 grams carbohydrate, 12 grams fat (39% of calories), 7 grams dietary fiber

1 burrito without cheese (estimate):
193 calories, 8 grams protein, 31 grams carbohydrate, 5 grams fat (23% of calories), 7 grams dietary fiber

SPLIT PEA SOUP
4 Servings

A family favorite, familiar to everyone. Surprisingly tasty—even without a ham bone!

Bring to a boil for 3 minutes, reduce heat and simmer until peas are tender—45 to 60 minutes:
6 cups water
1½ cups split peas, washed

Add and continue to simmer until vegetables are tender, 15 to 25 minutes, adding more water as needed:
½ cup chopped onion
2 fresh carrots, diced or sliced
3 stalks celery, chopped
1-2 teaspoons salt, to taste
1 bay leaf

Remove bay leaf. Puree part or all of soup in blender, if desired. This will help to thicken the soup.

Serve with:
Whole Wheat Popovers (p. 269), whole grain bread, or Minute Bran Muffins (p. 270)
Vegetable salad or vegetable relish tray

1½-cup serving:
290 calories, 19 grams protein, 52 grams carbohydrate, 1 gram fat (3% of calories), 10 grams dietary fiber

MIDDLE EASTERN LENTIL SOUP
4 to 6 Servings

Bring to a boil for 3 minutes, reduce heat and simmer (just below boiling) until lentils are tender, 30 to 60 minutes:
- **1½ cups lentils, washed**
- **7 cups water, vegetable or beef stock**
- **1 medium onion, chopped**
- **1 large or 2 medium stalks celery, chopped**
- **1 large or 2 medium carrots, diced**
- **1 clove garlic, minced**

Puree at least half the soup in blender and pour back into soup pot. Blend in:
- **3 tablespoons soy sauce, to taste**
- **juice of 1 lemon (or about 4 teaspoons)**
- **1 teaspoon cumin powder**
- **1 tablespoon butter**

Simmer 15 minutes longer. Add 5 to 10 minutes before serving:
- **½ cup minced fresh parsley**

Top each serving, if desired, with:
- **¼ cup grated cheddar or Jack cheese**

VARIATION:
—In place of soy sauce add 6 tablespoons Bragg Liquid Aminos (a health-food-store item lower in sodium and milder in flavor)

Serve with:
Pineapple Cornbread (p. 272) or rye bread or rye crackers
Vegetable munchies and dip

1-cup serving:
186 calories, 11.5 grams protein, 30 grams carbohydrate, 2.5 grams fat (12% of calories), 4.5 grams dietary fiber

SAVORY CHILI
8 Servings

Soak beans overnight in water:
2 cups dry kidney beans
8 cups water

Cover with water and freeze:
1 block tofu (12 to 19 oz.) (optional)

Bring beans and water to a boil for 10 minutes, reduce heat, and simmer until tender, about 2 to 3 hours. Add more water, if needed.

Place frozen tofu, if used, in a colander and thaw under running water; squeeze out excess water and crumble.

Sauté in a little olive oil:
1 onion, chopped
2 cups sliced fresh mushrooms
1 green pepper, chopped
2 cloves garlic, minced

Add to beans when tender:
2 15-oz. cans tomato sauce
  or 2 1-lb. cans tomato pieces
sautéed vegetables
crumbled tofu (optional)
1 tablespoon chili powder
1½ teaspoons cumin powder
1 teaspoon salt, to taste

Simmer 30 minutes longer to blend flavors.

Serve with:
Pineapple Cornbread (p. 272)
Carrot salad or carrot and celery sticks

1 serving (oil not included):
251 calories, 17 grams protein, 40 grams carbohydrate, 3.5 grams fat (13% of calories), 8 grams dietary fiber

CHILI
6 Servings

Make Savory Chili with the following changes:

Omit tofu.
Omit sautéed vegetables.

Add to cooked beans with tomato and seasonings:
1 chopped onion

Serve with:
Pineapple Cornbread (p. 272)
Carrot pineapple salad or carrot and celery sticks

1 serving:
269 calories, 16.5 grams protein, 50 grams carbohydrate, 1.5 grams fat (4% of calories), 9.5 grams dietary fiber

CREOLE BLACK-EYED PEAS 'N CORN
8 Servings

Soak 1 to 3 hours:
> **2 cups dry black-eyed peas**
> **8 cups water**

Sauté vegetables in butter:
> **2 tablespoons melted butter**
> **1 chopped onion**
> **1 chopped green pepper**

Bring peas in water to a boil and add:
> **sautéed vegetables**
> **1 bay leaf**
> **1 teaspoon Italian seasoning**
> **$1/2$ teaspoon rosemary**

Boil 3 minutes, reduce heat and simmer $1^1/2$ to 2 hours or until peas are tender. Add more water, if needed.

Add the following ingredients and simmer 30 minutes longer:
> **$1^1/2$ cups fresh or frozen corn**
> **16-oz. can stewed tomatoes**
> **8-oz. can tomato sauce**
> **$1/4$ cup ($1/2$ stick) butter**
> **2 tablespoons honey**
> **$1/2$ teaspoon salt**

Remove bay leaf before serving.

REDUCED FAT VARIATION:
—Sauté onion and pepper in only 1 tablespoon butter.
—Omit the $1/4$ cup butter. (The butter gives this dish a yummy flavor, but it is still a family favorite without it.)

Serve with:
Pineapple Cornbread (p. 272)
Carrot and celery sticks

1 serving:
296 calories, 12 grams protein, 42 grams carbohydrate, 9.5 grams fat (29% of calories), 6 grams dietary fiber

RATATOUILLE
4 Servings

Saute vegetables in fat until half-cooked:
> **2 tablespoons melted butter or olive oil**
> **1 coarsely chopped onion**
> **1 coarsely chopped green pepper**

Add and continue cooking until half-cooked:
> **1 small eggplant, unpeeled and coarsely chunked**
> **2 small zucchini, unpeeled and coarsely chunked**

Stir in:
> **2½ cups canned tomatoes**
> **½ teaspoon salt**
> **1 clove garlic, minced or ⅛ teaspoon garlic powder**
> **½ teaspoon sweet basil**

Bring to a boil, lower heat, and simmer about 5 minutes.

In separate container blend until smooth:
> **2 tablespoons cold water**
> **1 tablespoon arrowroot powder or cornstarch**

Blend mixture well into vegetables, stirring until lightly thickened, about 1 or 2 minutes.

Serve with Parmesan cheese, if desired.

LOW FAT VARIATION:
—Omit fat and "saute" vegetables in a little water.

Serve with:
Baked potato
Yellow vegetable
Coleslaw or tossed salad

1 serving:
159 calories, 5 grams protein, 24 grams carbohydrate, 2.5 grams fat (13% of calories), 7.5 grams dietary fiber

VEGETABLE LASAGNA
6 to 8 Servings

A refreshing no-wheat lasagna. A great company dish!

Wash, steam about 5 minutes until tender, and drain well. Chop and set aside:
   1 bunch fresh spinach

Sauté carrots, onions, garlic and mushrooms in olive oil:
   1 tablespoon olive oil
   ½ cup chopped onion
   1 cup diced carrots
   1 clove garlic, minced
   1 cup mushrooms, sliced (add during the last minute or two)

Blend into sautéed vegetables:
   2 cups tomato, pasta, or spaghetti sauce
   2¼-oz. can sliced ripe olives, drained
   1½ teaspoons oregano
   1 teaspoon sweet basil

While sauce simmers prepare:
   6 cups thin unpeeled zucchini slices (about 3 medium)
   ½ cup grated sharp cheddar cheese
   ½ cup grated mozzarella cheese

Mix together in another container:
   1 cup lowfat cottage cheese
   2 eggs
   ¼ cup Parmesan cheese

Layer ingredients in lightly greased 9" x 13" pan as follows:
   half the zucchini slices
   half the cottage cheese mixture
   half the spinach
   half the grated cheeses
   half the sauce mixture

Repeat the layers. Cover and bake at 375° for 30 minutes.

Serve with:
Fresh pineapple spears
Minute Bran Muffins (p. 270) or whole grain bread

1 serving (when 6 servings made):

309 calories, 19 grams protein, 18 grams carbohydrate, 12 grams fat (35% of calories), 13.5 grams dietary fiber

SWEET 'N SOUR TOFU STIR-FRY
6 Servings

Prepare in wok, if available.

Drain between paper towels on a plate for at least 30 minutes:
16 oz. block tofu

Meanwhile, prepare Sweet 'n Sour Sauce (p. 250).

Clean and cut Vegetables (p. 251).

In separate bowl blend together:
2 eggs
⅓ cup whole wheat flour
½ teaspoon salt (optional)

Cut drained tofu into 1" cubes and fold carefully into the egg-flour mixture to coat evenly. Brown coated tofu cubes on both sides until lightly browned in 2 tablespoons olive oil or without oil in non-stick pan; remove from pan.

Add 1 tablespoon oil to hot pan, or ⅓ cup water over medium-high heat. Add longer-cooking vegetables to pan and stir quickly. Cover with lid and cook about 2 minutes, stirring once. Add remaining vegetables, stirring quickly. Cover with lid and cook 2 to 5 minutes longer until just crisp-tender; stir a time or two.

Fold tofu cubes, Sweet 'n Sour Sauce, and pineapple reserved from making sauce into stir-fried vegetables and serve immediately.

Serve with:
Brown Rice (p. 226)
Leafy salad greens

1 serving with 1 cup vegetables (oil not included):

226 calories, 11 grams protein, 37 grams carbohydrate, 5.5 grams fat (22% of calories), 6.5 grams dietary fiber

SWEET 'N SOUR SAUCE
6 Servings

Drain juice into small saucepan and set pineapple chunks aside:
20-oz. can pineapple chunks, unsweetened
(about 1 cup pineapple juice)

Blend into juice with wire whisk:
⅓ cup apple cider vinegar
2 tablespoons arrowroot powder or cornstarch
2 tablespoons soy sauce
½ teaspoon ginger

Bring to a boil over medium heat, stirring constantly until thickened, about 1 minute. Add during last few seconds of cooking:
¼ cup honey

STIR-FRY VEGETABLES
(For Sweet 'n Sour Tofu Stir-Fry or Marinated Tofu Stir-Fry)

Cut any combination of vegetables, 1 to 2 cups per serving, into thin pieces and arrange on a platter; keep each vegetable separate or place shorter-cooking vegetables in bottom of a bowl and longer-cooking vegetables on top:

> **leafy greens such as spinach or chard,**
> **finely shredded**
> **water chestnuts, sliced**
> **zucchini, cut diagonally**
> **mushrooms, sliced**
> **green onion, chopped**
> **red or yellow onion, cut in rings**
> **green pepper, cut in thin strips**
> **cabbage, shredded**
> **broccoli—flowers cut in small pieces,**
> **stalks cut diagonally**
> **green beans, cut diagonally**
> **carrots, cut diagonally**
> **celery, cut diagonally**
> **cauliflower, small flowers**
> **bean sprouts**
> **peas, fresh or frozen**

Add 1 tablespoon oil to hot pan, or $1/3$ cup water over medium-high heat. Add longer-cooking vegetables to pan and stir quickly. Cover with lid and cook about 2 minutes, stirring once. Add shorter-cooking vegetables, stirring quickly. Cover with lid and cook 2 to 5 minutes longer until just crisp-tender; stir a time or two.

MARINATED TOFU STIR-FRY
6 Servings

To prepare the vegetables, follow Stir-Fry Vegetable preparation and cooking instructions on pages 249 and 251.

Drain between paper towels on a plate for at least 30 minutes:
16-oz. block regular or firm tofu

Meanwhile, blend together for marinade:
1/2 cup soy sauce
3 tablespoons lemon juice
2 teaspoons honey or granulated fructose
1 teaspoon ginger
1/8 teaspoon garlic powder

Cut tofu into 1" cubes and place in marinade for 1 hour or longer.

Brown cubes lightly in:
1 tablespoon oil or melted butter

Stir-fry vegetables and fold in tofu cubes.

VARIATION:
—Add cashews or almonds.

Serve with:
Brown rice and yogurt topping
Pineapple spears
Leafy salad greens

1 serving with 1 cup vegetables:
110 calories, 7.5 grams protein, 9 grams carbohydrate, 5.5 grams fat (45% of calories), 5.5 grams dietary fiber

TOFU SCRAMBLE
4 Servings

Drain thoroughly for at least 30 minutes between paper towels on large dinner plate:
16 oz. firm or regular tofu

Mash tofu coarsely with a fork on a clean, dry plate and place in mixing bowl. Blend into crumbled tofu:
2 tablespoons soy sauce
1/2 teaspoon dry mustard

Fold in:
4 fresh mushrooms, sliced
1 green onion, chopped
1 canned green chili, finely diced

Pour into non-stick fry pan, cover, and cook over medium heat about 15 minutes, or until slightly set.

Top with:
1/2 cup grated cheddar, Jack, or mozzarella cheese
Garnish with paprika

Serve, as desired, with:
ketchup
barbecue sauce
salsa

VARIATION:
—In place of soy sauce use 1/4 cup Bragg Liquid Aminos (a health-food-store item). It is lower in sodium and milder in flavor.

1 serving:
161 calories, 15 grams protein, 7 grams carbohydrate, 9.5 grams fat (53% of calories), 1 gram dietary fiber

LITTLE COTTAGE ENCHILADAS
4 Servings

Grate:
2 cups cheddar cheese

Set 1 cup of the cheese aside for topping and blend the other cup with:
1 cup lowfat cottage cheese
2 tablespoons chopped fresh parsley
1/2 teaspoon thyme
1/2 teaspoon marjoram
1/2 teaspoon oregano

In blender liquefy:
1/2 cup water
3 large outer leaves romaine lettuce
4-oz. can diced chilies, undrained

Simmer green sauce for 3 minutes in:
1 tablespoon melted butter

Pour 2/3 of the sauce in casserole dish.

Preheat oven to 400°.

In ungreased fry pan warm:
6 stoneground corn tortillas

Fill each tortilla with 1/3 cup cheese mixture and roll up. Place rolled tortillas in sauce in casserole dish, with edges tucked underneath. Pour remaining sauce over tortillas and top with:
remaining cup of cheddar cheese

Bake uncovered for 15 to 20 minutes at 400° until heated through and cheese melts.

Serve with:
Cooked carrots
Tomato-cucumber salad arranged on dark leafy greens
or vegetable relish tray

1 serving:
410 calories, 24 grams protein, 27 grams carbohydrate, 24.5 grams fat (52% of calories), 0.5 grams dietary fiber

FETTUCCINE
4 Servings

Combine and bring to a boil:
4 quarts water
¼ teaspoon salt

Add and boil 5 to 6 minutes until tender (Do not overcook!):
8 oz. whole grain noodles

Drain and rinse in cool water.

Sauté almonds and garlic in butter:
¼ cup melted butter
¼ cup chopped or slivered almonds
2 cloves garlic, minced

Blend into almonds and garlic:
1 cup sour cream
½ cup Parmesan cheese
1 teaspoon salt, to taste

Fold in and heat to serving temperature:
cooked, drained noodles
¼ cup finely chopped fresh parsley

1 serving:
529 calories, 19 grams protein, 43 grams carbohydrate, 32 grams fat (54% of calories), 5 grams dietary fiber

REDUCED FAT VARIATION:
—Replace half the sour cream with nonfat yogurt or use light sour cream (Knutsen Nice 'n Light); omit sautéing almonds and garlic in butter.

Serve with:
Green or yellow vegetable
Tossed salad

1 serving reduced fat variation:
383 calories, 19 grams protein, 45 grams carbohydrate, 14.5 grams fat (34% of calories), 5 grams dietary fiber

TUNA NOODLE YUMMY
6 Servings

Follow recipe for Fettuccine (p. 255).

With the almonds and garlic sauté:
½ cup chopped celery
½ cup chopped onion

Fold into sauce with noodles and parsley and heat to serving temperature:
6½-oz. can water-packed tuna sprinkled with
1 teaspoon lemon juice
½ cup frozen peas

1 serving:

758 calories, 23 grams protein, 32 grams carbohydrates, 2.15 grams fat (25% of calories), 5 grams dietary fiber

REDUCED FAT VARIATION:
—Replace half the sour cream with nonfat yogurt or use light sour cream (Knutsen Nice 'n Light); omit sautéing in butter; omit almonds.

Serve with:
Yellow vegetable
Spinach or green salad

1 serving reduced fat version:

632 calories, 22 grams protein, 32 grams carbohydrate, 7 grams fat (10% of calories), 5 grams dietary fiber

TARTAR SAUCE
7/8 Cup

Blend together until smooth with wire whisk:
   3/4 cup nonfat or lowfat plain yogurt
   2 tablespoons mayonnaise
   1 teaspoon lemon juice
   1/8 teaspoon onion powder
   1/8 teaspoon salt (optional)

VARIATIONS:
—Add 1/2 teaspoon Health Valley Fish Herb Seasoning.
—Add chopped dill pickle or honey-sweetened or unsweetened
   pickle relish (from a health food store).

1 serving (1 tablespoon):
22 calories, 0.5 gram protein, no carbohydrate, 1.5 grams fat (65% of calories), no dietary fiber

LEMON BAKED FISH
4 to 6 Servings

A good recipe for lean fish. Purchase 6 oz. fish fillet or 8 oz. steak per person of halibut, cod, fillet of sole, or any other lean fish.

In bottom of baking pan melt at low heat in oven:
¼ cup butter

Remove pan from oven and turn oven to 350° to preheat. Place in single layer in buttered pan:
fish fillets or steaks

Spoon some of the butter over the top.

Squeeze over the top of the fish:
juice of 1 lemon (about 4 teaspoons)

Lightly sprinkle with:
salt or Health Valley Fish Herb Seasoning
paprika
fresh minced or dried parsley flakes

Bake uncovered for 20 to 30 minutes until fish is tender, basting 1 or 2 times. Fish is done when it flakes easily with a fork and the translucent flesh has turned opaque. Do not overcook!

1 serving (6 oz.):

231 calories, 32.5 grams protein, 1 gram carbohydrate, 10 grams fat (38% of calories), no fiber

REDUCED FAT VARIATION:
—Omit butter.
—Lay fish in a non-stick pan sprayed with Pam spray.
—Add a couple tablespoons of water.
—Cover tightly to bake, basting 2 or 3 times.

Serve with:
Baked potato or brown rice
Green vegetable
Carrot-raisin salad

1 serving (6 oz.):

164 calories, 32.5 grams protein, 1 gram carbohydrate, 2.5 grams fat (12% of calories), no fiber

BAKED SALMON
4 to 6 Servings

Good for any fat fish such as bluefish, herring, mackerel, pompano, whitefish, salmon, mullet, and sablefish.

Follow Lemon Baked Fish recipe (p. 258), reducing butter to 1 tablespoon.

Do not cover while baking.

Serve with:
Baked potato or brown rice
Garden patch salad (shredded carrot, chopped celery, cucumber, tomato, cauliflowerettes, frozen peas, green onion, choice of dressing)

1 serving (6 oz.):
323 calories, 33 grams protein, no carbohydrate, 18 grams fat (50% of calories)

BAKED PARMESAN CHICKEN
6 5.3-oz. Servings

A gourmet favorite for company and banquets!

Melt in baking pan at about 250°:
   ½ cup (1 stick) butter

Meanwhile, mix together in blender until small bread crumbs are formed:
   1 slice whole wheat bread or amount needed to make about 1 cup soft crumbs, not packed
   2 or 3 sprigs fresh parsley to make about ¼ cup minced
   ½ cup Parmesan cheese
   ⅛ teaspoon garlic powder
   ⅛ teaspoon salt

Remove skin and visible fat from chicken:
   2 lbs. boneless chicken breast pieces

Remove melted butter from oven and coat chicken first in the butter, then with crumb mixture. Lay chicken in remaining butter in pan, top with any remaining crumb mixture, sprinkle with paprika if desired, and bake uncovered at 350° until tender, about 1 hour.

Baste chicken a time or two during baking. Cover with foil if coating starts to brown too much before chicken is tender.

1 serving:

491 calories, 52.5 grams protein, 5 grams carbohydrate, 26.5 grams fat (49% of calories), 0.5 grams dietary fiber

REDUCED FAT VARIATION:
—Reduce Parmesan cheese to 3 tablespoons.
—Omit butter; bake in non-stick pan or pan coated with Pam spray.
—Dip coated chicken pieces in nonfat milk, as needed, in place of melted butter.

Serve with:
Brown Rice (p. 226) or Brown Rice Pilaf (p. 227)
Green or yellow vegetable
Tossed salad

1 serving:

344 calories, 51.5 grams protein, 6 grams carbohydrate, 10 grams fat (10% of calories), 0.5 gram dietary fiber

CASHEW CHICKEN
4 to 6 Servings

Serve without sauce, if desired.

Cook:
> **2 cups chopped chicken**

Skin and chop boneless breast, cover with water, and bring to a boil. Reduce heat and simmer 30 minutes or until tender; set aside.

Blend together for sauce and set aside:
> **1 cup pineapple juice**
> **2 tablespoons soy sauce**
> **2 tablespoons arrowroot powder or cornstarch**
> **1/2 teaspoon ginger**

Sauté vegetables in oil until crisp-tender (about 4 minutes):
> **1 tablespoon olive oil**
> **2 cups celery, sliced thinly on diagonal**
> **1 medium onion, sliced**

Add and cook another minute or two:

> **1/2 cup fresh or frozen green peas or 1 bunch steamed, chopped spinach**
> **1 red bell pepper cut in strips or small jar pimento strips**

Blend in sauce; cook and stir to thicken.

Fold in and heat thoroughly:
> **2 cups cooked diced chicken**
> **1/2 cup unsalted cashews**
> **1 cup fresh pineapple chunks**

VARIATION:
—Use 20-oz. can unsweetened pineapple chunks, draining the juice for the sauce.

Serve with:
Brown rice or whole wheat noodles
Yellow vegetable
Leafy salad greens

1 serving (when 4 servings made):

359 calories, 27.5 grams protein, 28 grams carbohydrate, 16 grams fat (40% of calories), 6 grams dietary fiber

CHICKEN CHOP SUEY
4 to 6 Servings

Place chicken in a pot and bring slowly to a boil. Reduce heat and cook until chicken is tender:
> **2¹/₂ lb. chicken, skinned**
> **water to cover well**
> **a little chopped onion, celery, and carrot**

Drain, saving broth; cool chicken, remove bones; set aside.

Chop vegetables:
> **2 cups celery, thinly sliced on diagonal**
> **2 cups shredded napa (Chinese) cabbage**
> **2 cups bok choy, shredded**
> **1 onion, chopped**

Bring to a boil and reduce heat to simmer:
> **2 cups chicken broth**
> **1¹/₂ teaspoons granulated fructose or honey**
> **¹/₄ cup soy sauce**

Add celery and onions to broth; simmer about 10 to 15 minutes. Add remaining vegetables and cook about 5 minutes longer.

Blend together separately and stir into broth, continuing to stir constantly until thickened:
> **¹/₄ cup cold water**
> **2¹/₂ tablespoons arrowroot powder or cornstarch**

Add chicken with:
> **8-oz. can sliced water chestnuts, drained**
> **¹/₂ teaspoon salt, to taste**

Serve with:
Brown Rice (p. 226)
Orange and pineapple slices on leafy green lettuce

1 serving (when 6 servings made):
178 calories, 17.5 grams protein, 19 grams carbohydrate, 4.5 grams fat (22% of calories), 6 grams dietary fiber

CASHEW CHOP SUEY
4 to 6 Servings

Follow recipe for Chicken Chop Suey (p. 262). Omit chicken. Use water in place of chicken broth for vegetarian dish, if desired.

Add just before serving:
   ½ to ¾ cup unsalted cashews

Serve with:
Brown Rice (p. 226).
Orange and pineapple slices on leafy green lettuce

1 serving (when 6 servings made and ¾ cup cashews used):

184 calories, 6.5 grams protein, 24 grams carbohydrate, 9.5 grams fat (47% of calories), 6 grams dietary fiber

COOKED BROCCOLI
1 lb. per 3 to 4 Servings

A fool-proof method!

Bring to a boil enough water to cover broccoli.

Add broccoli gradually to the water so that it continues to boil; boil uncovered for 40-60 seconds—no longer! Drain (save water for soup, if desired).

Broccoli cooked by this method holds its texture and color well if kept hot in a covered pan in the oven until ready to serve, or chilled in refrigerator for use in a salad the next day.

1 serving (1 cup):

40 calories, 5 grams protein, 7 grams carbohydrate, 0.5 gram fat (11% of calories), 9 grams dietary fiber, 3900 IU carotene (provitamin A), 140 mg. vitamin C, 140 mg. calcium, 410 mg. potassium, 16 mg. sodium

STEAMED BROCCOLI

Place broccoli in vegetable steamer basket over boiling water and cook 2 minutes uncovered. Cover and cook until crisp-tender, about 5-10 minutes.

1 serving (1 cup):
40 calories, 5 grams protein, 7 grams carbohydrate, 0.5 gram fat (11% of calories), 9 grams dietary fiber, 3900 IU carotene (provitamin A), 140 mg. vitamin C, 140 mg. calcium, 410 mg. potassium, 16 mg. sodium

ALMOND TUNA SALAD
2 Servings

Mix together:
>   **6.5-oz. can water-packed tuna, well drained**
>   **¼ cup nonfat plain yogurt**
>   **2 tablespoons mayonnaise**
>   **2 teaspoons lemon juice**
>   **1 stalk celery, chopped**
>   **1 slice onion, chopped**
>   **⅓ cup chopped or slivered almonds**

Arrange on each individual salad plate in the following order:
>   **leaf of green leafy lettuce**
>   **2 cups broken leafy and iceberg lettuce**
>   **1 tomato, cut almost through in wedges to form**
>   **a tomato "flower"**
>   **half the tuna almond mixture mounded in center**
>   **of tomato "flower"**
>   **Garnish paprika on tuna mixture**
>   **Ripe olive in center of tuna mixture**

Garnish with parsley sprigs.

Serve with:
Whole grain muffins or rolls
Carrot sticks and cucumber slices

1 serving:

403 calories, 35.5 grams protein, 13 grams carbohydrate, 23 grams fat (51% of calories), 0.5 gram dietary fiber

TOFU SALAD SPREAD
About 3 Cups

Especially tasty with whole wheat pita breads or on whole wheat sandwich bread.

Drain between paper towels on a plate for at least 30 minutes:
  16-oz. block regular or firm tofu

Mash drained tofu with a fork and blend in:
  $1/2$ cup finely chopped onion
     or 2 tablespoons instant chopped onion
  2 celery stalks, finely chopped
  $1/4$ cup chopped green pepper
  $1/4$ cup mayonnaise
  1 to 2 tablespoons apple cider vinegar, to taste
  2 teaspoons prepared mustard
  $1/2$ teaspoon garlic powder
  $1/4$ teaspoon tumeric (for yellow color)

$1/4$ cup serving:
71 calories, 3 grams protein, 2 grams carbohydrate, 5.5 grams fat (72% of calories), 0.5 gram dietary fiber

SUNSHINE SHAKE
1 Serving

Wake up your day or pick up your day with this satisfying tasty potassium-and-vitamin-C-rich drink!

Blend together until smooth in the blender:
1 medium orange, peeled and cut in chunks
1 medium banana, peeled
½ cup lowfat or nonfat plain yogurt
    or lowfat vanilla yogurt
¹⁄₁₆ teaspoon nutmeg
¹⁄₁₆ teaspoon cinnamon

1 serving (with lowfat vanilla yogurt):

271 calories, 10 grams protein, 61 grams carbohydrate, 2.5 grams fat (8% of calories), 5 grams dietary fiber

WHOLE WHEAT POPOVERS
Makes 12 Large

Great with soups! Serve hot immediately after baking.

Preheat oven to 450°.
Grease muffin pan very well (a muffin pan with deeper cups is best).

Mix together in blender on high speed about 30 seconds:
3 large eggs
1½ cups lowfat milk
1 cup whole wheat pastry flour
¾ teaspoon salt

Pour batter evenly into muffin cups, filling at least ¾ full.

Bake at 450° for 15 minutes; turn heat down to 350° and continue baking about 20 minutes until golden. Cool 5 minutes before removing from pan. Serve immediately.

Do not expect these to rise as high as white flour popovers! Do not be surprised if popovers fall in the middle—they are hollow inside.

Delicious with butter or jam.

1 popover:
80 calories, 4 grams protein, 11 grams carbohydrate, 2.5 grams fat (25% of calories), 1 gram dietary fiber

MINUTE BRAN MUFFINS
10 to 12 Large

These go with everything! Serve warm or cold.

Preheat oven to 350°. Grease muffin pan or line with muffin papers.

Cover with warm water and let stand 5 to 10 minutes:
    ½ cup raisins (optional)

Blend together and let stand for 5 minutes:
    ½ cup boiling water
    1½ cups unprocessed wheat bran (Miller's)

Blend together thoroughly with wire whisk in order given:
    1 egg
    ¼ to ⅓ cup honey
    1 cup buttermilk or sour milk
    bran mixture

Blend dry ingredients together in separate bowl:
    1½ cups whole wheat or whole wheat pastry flour
    1¼ teaspoons soda
    1 teaspoon salt
    ½ cup walnuts, chopped (optional)

Blend drained raisins, then dry ingredients into liquid ingredients just until mixed. Do not overmix! Fill muffin cups almost full. Fill any empty cups halfway with water. Bake 20 to 25 minutes at 350°. Cool 5 to 10 minutes before removing from pan.

---

1 muffin (when 10 muffins made)—raisins/walnuts not included:

145 calories, 4.5 grams protein, 32 grams carbohydrate, 1.5 grams fat (11% of calories), 6 grams dietary fiber

EMILIE'S DELUXE BRAN MUFFINS
12 Large

Follow recipe for Minute Bran Muffins using:
- **1 cup chopped dates or date dices**
- **1 cup raisins**
- **1 cup chopped walnuts**
- **1 cup shredded coconut, unsweetened (optional)**

1 muffin (coconut not included):

263 calories, 6 grams protein, 58 grams carbohydrate, 7.5 grams fat (26% of calories), 7 grams dietary fiber

PINEAPPLE CORNBREAD
12 servings

Preheat oven to 350°.

Blend together:
> **2 eggs**
> **2 tablespoons honey**
> **20-oz. can unsweetened crushed pineapple, undrained**

Blend dry ingredients thoroughly in separate bowl:
> **3 cups stoneground cornmeal**
> **2 teaspoons baking powder**
> **1 teaspoon salt**

Blend liquid ingredients into dry ingredients just until mixed. Pour into greased 8″ or 9″ square pan. Bake 25 to 35 minutes.

VARIATIONS:
—In place of 1 cup cornmeal use 1 cup whole wheat flour.
—Add 4 tablespoons melted butter or oil (or less). Increases fat per piece to 6 grams (28% of calories).

1 piece (12 per recipe):
161 calories, 4 grams protein, 29 grams carbohydrate, 2 grams fat (13% of calories), 4.5 grams dietary fiber

PINEAPPLE SUNSHINE MOLD
8 to 10 Servings

Stir gelatin into juice to soften and let stand 5 minutes:
   3/4 cup orange juice
   1 package (2 teaspoons) unflavored gelatin

Meanwhile, mix together in mixing bowl:
   8-oz. can crushed pineapple, undrained
   6-oz. can unsweetened pineapple juice
   1 orange, peeled and chopped
   1 banana, sliced
   1/4 cup chopped pecans or almonds (optional)

Heat gelatin mixture over medium heat, stirring constantly until gelatin is dissolved. Remove from heat and blend in:
   3 tablespoons honey

Add gelatin mixture to remaining ingredients. Pour into 8" or 9" square pan or a 9" x 13" pan and chill until set.

Cut into squares for individual servings and garnish as desired with mint leaves, whole strawberries, and yogurt-sour cream topping (half and half).

1 serving (when 8 servings made per recipe)—garnish not included:

114 calories, 2.5 grams protein, 29 grams carbohydrate, negligible fat, 1.5 grams dietary fiber

FROZEN VANILLA YOGURT
2 Cups

Incredibly easy to make, low calorie and low fat!

Liquefy in blender:
2 cups nonfat or lowfat plain yogurt
¼ cup granulated fructose
1 teaspoon vanilla

Pour into bowl or ice tray and freeze till set. Scoop into electric mixer and beat until soft. Place beaten mixture into the blender and liquefy, if desired (this will increase the creaminess). Refreeze until set.

Allow to stand at room temperature about 10 minutes before serving.

½ cup serving:
140 calories, 7 grams protein, 23 grams carbohydrate, 2.5 grams fat (16% of calories), no fiber

EMILIE'S YUMMY OATMEALS
4 Dozen

These rich and delectable cookies are chock-full of nutritious goodies!

Cream together:
> ½ **cup soft butter (oil may be used)**
> ⅔ **cup honey**

Blend in:
> **1 egg**

Blend dry ingredients in separate bowl:
> **1 cup whole wheat pastry flour**
> **or whole wheat flour**
> **1 teaspoon cinnamon**
> **½ teaspoon soda**
> **½ teaspoon salt**
> **¼ teaspoon nutmeg**

Stir dry ingredients by hand into creamed ingredients just until mixed (do not overmix).

Blend in by hand just until mixed:
> **2 cups rolled oats, uncooked**
> **1 cup raisins**
> **1 cup carob chips**
> **1 cup chopped dates or date dices**
> **1 cup chopped walnuts**

Drop by spoonfuls onto greased cookie sheets. If dough does not seem to hold together well, press each spoonful together a bit with fingertips after filling up the cookie sheet.

Bake at 350° for 10 to 12 minutes. Cool before removing from cookie sheets.

VARIATION:
—Add 1 cup medium shred or macaroon shred unsweetened coconut (doesn't change nutrient amounts much).

1 cookie:
109 calories, 2 grams protein, 23 grams carbohydrate, 5 grams fat (39% of calories), 1.5 grams dietary fiber

EMILIE'S OLIVE OIL DRESSING
1³/₄ Cups

Mash together with tip of a knife and put in pint jar:
3 cloves garlic, pressed
1 teaspoon salt
¹/₂ scant teaspoon pepper

Add and shake well; chill:
1 cup olive oil
¹/₂ cup wine vinegar
juice of 1 lemon (about ¹/₄ cup)

1 tablespoon serving:

69 calories, 9 grams fat (100% of calories)

SUE'S HOUSE DRESSING
1½ Cups

Blend thoroughly with wire whisk:
  1 cup nonfat or lowfat plain yogurt
  ½ cup mayonnaise
  1 tablespoon lemon juice
  1 teaspoon fresh or dry parsley or chives
  ½ teaspoon onion powder
  ¼ teaspoon salt (optional)
  ⅛ teaspoon garlic powder

1 tablespoon serving:
39 calories, 4 grams fat (87% of calories)

THOUSAND ISLAND DRESSING
2½ Cups

Blend thoroughly with wire whisk:
   1¼ cups nonfat plain yogurt
   ¾ cup mayonnaise
   ¼ cup ketchup
   1 tablespoon lemon juice
   1½ teaspoons granulated fructose
   ¼ teaspoon salt
   ⅛ teaspoon garlic powder
   1 small dill pickle, chopped fine or honey sweetened pickle relish

1 tablespoon serving:
34 calories, 3.5 grams fat (89% of calories)

Notes

Chapter 6

1. *Understanding Vitamins and Minerals: The Prevention Total Health System*, editors of *Prevention Magazine* (Emmaus, PA: Rodale Press, 1984), p. 6.

Chapter 7

1. Percentage losses adapted from: Ethel Renwick, *Let's Try Real Food* (Grand Rapids, MI: Zondervan Publishing House, 1976), p. 29, and Audrey Eyton, *The F-Plan Diet* (New York: Crown Publishers, 1973), pp. 79-80.

Chapter 11

1. Bonnie Liebman, "Burgerland Revisited," *Nutrition Action Healthletter*, 12:5 (Washington, DC: Center for Science in the Public Interest, June 1985), p. 1.

Chapter 16

1. "Is Fat More Fattening?" *Diet & Nutrition Letter*, 4:12 (New York: Tufts University, Feb. 1987), p. 2.

Chapter 18

1. Warren N. Levin, "What's the Story on Fats?" *Your Health* (Overland Park, KS: International Academy of Preventive Medicine, Jan. 1984), p. 1.
2. "More Superfoods," *Nutrition News*, 4:12 (Pomona, CA, 1981), p. 1.
3. Kerry Pechter, "The Amazing Benefits of the New Fiber Supplements," *Prevention Magazine* (Emmaus, PA: Rodale Press, Oct. 1982), p. 27.

Chapter 19

1. "4 to 10 Chickens on Market Contaminated, Says USDA," *Press-Enterprise* (Riverside County, CA, Feb. 18, 1987), p. A-1.
2. "U.S.A. 1971-1983 Estimated Association With Salmonella Illnesses," distributed by Raymond A. Novell, attorney for Alta-Dena Dairy (1085 West Badillo, Covina, CA 91722).

3. Elaine Blume, "Germ Wars," *Nutrition Action Healthletter,*Vol. 13:6 (Washington, DC: Center for Science in the Public Interest, June 1986), p. 4.
4. John A. Scharffenberg, *Problems With Meat* (Santa Barbara, CA: Woodbridge Press Publishing Company, 1979), p. 33.
5. Gary Null, *The New Vegetarian* (New York: William Morrow and Company, 1978), p. 19.

Chapter 20

1. Gladys Lindberg and Judy Lindberg McFarland, *Take Charge of Your Health* (San Francisco: Harper & Row Publishers, 1982), pp. 79-80.
2. "Hold the Eggs and Butter," *Time* (Mar. 26, 1984), p. 58.
3. Ibid., p. 58.
4. Null, *The New Vegetarian*, p. 121.
5. Lindberg, *Take Charge of Your Health*, p. 80.

Chapter 21

1. Null, *The New Vegetarian*, p. 89.
2. Bernard Jensen, "Raw Milk Vs. Pasteurized Milk," *Health Freedom News* (National Health Federation, May 1985), p. 41 and "Which Do You Choose?" Alta-Dena Dairy printed brochure.
3. Frances M. Pottenger, Jr., "The Effect of Heat-Processed Foods and Metabolized Vitamin D Milk on the Dentofacial Structures of Experimental Animals" (Reprinted from *American Journal of Orthodontics and Oral Surgery,* St. Louis, Vol. 32, No. 8, Oral Surgery pages 467-85, Aug. 1946), p. 9.
4. Jensen, *Health Freedom News*, p. 41.
5. "U.S.A. 1971-1983 Estimated Association With Salmonella Illnesses," distributed by Raymond A. Novell, attorney for Alta-Dena Dairy (1085 West Badillo, Covina, CA 91722).
6. "Hold the Eggs and Butter," p. 62.
7. S. I. McMillen, *None of These Diseases* (Charlotte, NC: Commission Press, 1979), pp. 14-16.
8. Weston A. Price, *Nutrition and Physical Degeneration* (La Mesa, CA: The Price-Pottenger Nutrition Foundation, 1970), p. 291.

Chapter 23

1. "Why Sugar Continues to Concern Nutritionists," *Diet & Nutrition Letter,* Vol. 3, No. 3 (New York: Tufts University, May 1985), p. 3.
2. "Book Shelf," *Better Nutrition* (Atlanta: Communications Channels, Inc., Oct. 1984), p. 35.
3. "Sugar and Breast Cancer," *Better Nutrition* (Atlanta: Communications Channels, Inc., July 1983), pp. 13-14ff.

4. Frances Sheridan Goulart, "Sugar Substitutes," *The Herbalist* (Nov. 1979), p. 21.

Chapter 25

1. Ruth Adams, "Does Excessive Salt Cause High Blood Pressure?" *Better Nutrition* (Atlanta: Communications Channels, Inc., May 1985), p. 23.
2. Adams, *Better Nutrition*, p. 23.
3. Adams, *Better Nutrition*, p. 37.

Chapter 26

1. Bonnie F. Liebman, "Fated to Be Fat?" *Nutrition Action Healthletter* (Washington, DC: Center for Science in the Public Interest, Jan./Feb. 1987), p. 1.

Chapter 29

1. Bernard Fensterwald, III, NNF Legislative Counsel, "Washington Watch—Fighting Crime With Nutrition," *Health Food Review* (Apr. 1983), p. 72.

Chapter 33

1. Ruth Bircher, *Eating Your Way to Health* (London: Faber and Faber, 1961), pp. 32-33.
2. Letitia Brewster and Michael Jacobson, *The Changing American Diet* (Washington, DC: Center for Science in the Public Interest, 1983), p. 1.
3. Elaine Blume and Michael F. Jacobson, "Food Irradiation: Is the Time Ripe?" *Nutrition Action Healthletter* (Washington, DC: Center for Science in the Public Interest, Nov. 1986), p. 7.

Chapter 34

1. John White, *Masks of Melancholy,* (Downers Grove, IL: InterVarsity Press, 1982), p. 41.
2. White, *Masks of Melancholy,* p. 42.

Chapter 35

1. *The Relation of Christian Faith to Health*, adopted by the 172nd General Assembly, May 1960 (The United Presbyterian Church in the United States of America, Board of National Missions, 475 Riverside Drive, New York, NY 10027), p. 39.
2. *The Relation of Christian Faith to Health*, p. 38.

Chapter 36

1. *The Relation of Christian Faith to Health,* Adopted by the 172nd General Assembly, May 1960 (The United Presbyterian Church in the United States of America, Board of National Missions, 475 Riverside Drive, New York, NY 10027), p. 39.
2. *The Relation of Christian Faith to Health,* p. 56.

Chapter 37

1. Dr. Hans Diehl, *To Your Health* (Redlands, CA: The Quiet Hour, 1987), p. 190.
2. Lindberg, *Take Charge of Your Health,* p. 14.

Chapter 38

1. *The Higher Taste* (based on the teachings of A. C. Bhaktivedanta Swami Prabhupada, founder of the International Society for Krishna Consciousness (Los Angeles: The Bhaktivedanta Book Trust, 1984), p. 52.
2. Ibid., p. 51.
3. Ibid., p. 51.
4. Ibid., p. 52.
5. Ibid., p. 53.
6. Ibid., p. 52.
7. Ibid., p. 52.
8. Ibid., p. 52.
9. Ibid., p. 53.

Chapter 39

1. Carol McGraw, "Seekers of Self Now Herald the 'New Age,' " *Los Angeles Times* (Feb. 17, 1987), p. I-17.
2. McGraw, *Los Angeles Times,* p. 16.
3. McGraw, *Los Angeles Times,* p. 16.
4. Laurel Robertson, Carol Flinders, and Bronwen Godfrey, *Laurel's Kitchen* (Berkeley, CA: Nilgiri Press, 1976), p. 46.

Chapter 43

1. Robert Van Treeck, Jr., "In Other Worlds," *U Magazine* (Downers Grove, IL: Inter-Varsity Christian Fellowship, Feb. 1987), p. 10.
2. Frances Moore Lappe, *Diet For a Small Planet,* Tenth Anniversary Edition (New York: Ballantine Books, 1982), p. 152.
3. Daniel Doriani, "Wasn't The Lord's Supper Originally a Feast?" *Christianity Today,* Mar. 18, 1983, p. 44.

Chapter 44

1. D.B. Jelliffe, "Commerciogenic Malnutrition?" *Nutritional Reviews*, 30:9, (Sep. 1972), p. 43.

Chapter 45

1. Keith Green, lyrics from "So You Wanna Go Back to Egypt?" (Sparrow Records, Inc.).

Recommended Reading

Additives

King, C. D. *What's That You're Eating?!!* Newport Beach, CA: C. D. King Ltd., 1982.

Allergies

Cocoa, Arthur F. *The Pulse Test. (Easy Allergy Detection)* New York: Arco Publishing Company, 1979.
Crook, William G. *Tracking Down Hidden Food Allergy.* Jackson, TN: Professional Books, 1980.
Ludeman, Kate and Henderson, Louise. *Do-It-Yourself Allergy Analysis Handbook.* New Cannon, CT: Keats Publishing, 1979.
Mandell, Marshall and Scanlon, Lynne. *Dr. Mandell's Five-Day Allergy Relief System.* New York, NY: Pocket Books, 1979.

Biblical Health Standards

McMillen, S.I. *None of These Diseases.* Old Tappan, NJ: Fleming H. Revell Company, 1983.

Children, Teaching

Gooch, Sandy. *If You Love Me, Don't Feed Me Junk!* Reston, VA: Reston Publishing Company, Inc., 1983.

Exercise

Frank, Marge and Linton, Nancy, *The Better Better Body Book.* Grand Rapids, MI: Zondervan Publishing House, 1985.

Family Relationships

Littauer, Florence. *How To Get Along With Difficult People.* Eugene, OR: Harvest House Publishers, 1984.
Littauer, Florence. *Personality Plus.* Old Tappan, NJ: Fleming H. Revell Company, 1983.

Littauer, Florence. *Your Personality Tree*. Waco, TX: Word Books, 1986.

Fasting

Omartian, Stormie. *Greater Health God's Way*. Canoga Park, CA: Sparrow Press, 1984.

Smith, Harold J. *Fast Your Way to Health*. Nashville, TN: Thomas Nelson Publishers, 1975.

Wallis, Arthur. *God's Chosen Fast*. Ft. Washington, PA: Christian Literature Crusade, 1974.

Food Safety

Null, Gary. *The New Vegetarian*. New York, NY: William Morrow and Company, Inc., 1978.

Samsidis, Nicholas. *Homogenized!* Glenwood Landing, NY: Sunflower Publishing, Inc., 1983.

Oster, Kurt A. and Ross, Donald J. *The XO Factor*. New York: Park City Press, 1983.

Food Storage

Bailey, Janet. *Keeping Food Fresh*. Garden City, NY: The Dial Press, 1985.

General Health

Omartian, Stormie. *Greater Health God's Way: Seven Steps To Health, Youthfulness and Vitality*. Canoga Park, CA: Sparrow Press, 1984.

Human Body

Brand, Paul and Yancey, Phillip. *Fearfully and Wonderfully Made*. Grand Rapids, MI: Zondervan Publishing House, 1980.

Brand, Paul and Yancey, Phillip. *In His Image*. Grand Rapids, MI: Zondervan Publishing House, 1984.

Jewish Feasts for Christian Celebration

Zimmerman, Martha. *Celebrate The Feasts*. Minneapolis, MN: Bethany House Publishers, 1975.

Shopping

Goldbeck, Nikki and Goldbeck, David. *The Supermarket Handbook*. New York: New American Library, 1976.

Therapeutic Diets

Airola, Paavo. *How To Get Well*. Arizona: Health Plus Publishers, 1974.

Vitamins/Minerals

Nutrition Search, Inc. *Nutrition Almanac*. New York: McGraw-Hill Book Co., 1979.

Weight

Katahn, Martin. *Beyond Diet*. New York: Berkley Books, 1984.

World Effects of the Western Diet

Price, Weston A. *Nutrition and Physical Degeneration*. La Mesa, CA: The Price Pottenger Nutrition Foundation, 1970. (Available by mail; order brochure: P.O. Box 2624, La Mesa, CA 92041.)

World Hunger (Request information and book list)

Institute of Food and Development Policy, 1885 Mission Street, San Francisco, CA 94103-3584.

Resources from the Authors

For more information regarding speaking engagements and additional materials on personal, kitchen, household, and holiday organization, please address all correspondence to:

> Bob & Emilie Barnes
> MORE HOURS IN MY DAY
> 2838 Rumsey Drive
> Riverside, CA 92506
>
> (Enclose 2 first-class stamps)

For more information regarding speaking engagements, the *Eating Better Cookbooks* (Main Dish, Muffins, Soups, Breakfast, Lunches and Snacks, Desserts, Yeast Breads), *Eating Better with Sue* video, and newsletter, please address all correspondence to:

> Rich & Sue Gregg
> EATING BETTER WITH SUE
> 8830 Glencoe Drive
> Riverside, CA 92503
>
> (Enclose 2 first-class stamps)